Marcy & Jorry

with all my love!

GUT HELP

GUIDE TO BREAKING FREE OF IBD AND IBS

GUT HELP
GUIDE TO BREAKING FREE OF IBD AND IBS

By Stephen Demirjian

MAHAMA PUBLISHING

Publisher's Cataloging-In-Publication Data
(Prepared by The Donohue Group, Inc.)

Demirjian, Stephen.
  Gut help : guide to breaking free of IBD and IBS / by Stephen Demirjian. --
1st ed.

    p. ; cm.

    ISBN-13: 978-0-9786673-0-6
    ISBN-10: 0-9786673-0-1

1. Inflammatory bowel diseases--Popular works. 2. Colitis--Popular works. 3. Colitis--Alternative treatment. 4. Crohn's disease--Popular works. 5. Crohn's disease--Alternative treatment. 6. Irritable colon--Popular works. I. Title.

RC862.I53 D46 2006
616.3/44   2006928501

Mahama books are available for special promotions, premiums, educational and fund raising needs. For details, contact Mahama Publishing. info@mahamapub.com

Cover Design and Layout by Elaine Devine, Devine Design, 19 Old Stagecoach Drive, Monson, MA 01057

Photography by James A. Langone, James A. Langone Photography, Inc., 36 Loring Street, Springfield, MA 01108. Back cover baseball photo by Terry Pellerin

FIRST EDITION

IMPORTANT NOTICE TO READERS

ACKNOWLEDGEMENTS

This book would not have been possible if it weren't for the infinite love and support of my immediate family: my father, Harry, for getting this whole thing started and for all his scientific research, experience, and care; my mother, Ellie, for her boundless positivity, sensitivity, and expert cooking lessons; my brother Andrew, sister Ali and sister-in-law Dahlia for their undying support and constant comic relief. Maria Torres for being there for me when I started this whole journey. And the rest of my family, the Tevans, Hachigians, Colombosians and Demirjians for their endless support, laughs and love.

I would also like to thank my wonderful editors, Dahlia Elsayed and Harry Demirjian, your comments and insights magically turned this daunting task into something doable. Charles Demirjian, Esq., and Jay Hachigian, Esq. for legal counsel and guidance. My fantastic graphic designer, Elaine Devine at Devine Design, a million thank-yous for all your experience and hard work. Jim Langone for going along with my crazy ideas for the photo shoot. Kenny "Janik" Janjigian for being a great listener and loving dog sitter during some tough times. Scout Stevenson for sage tech advice. Christopher Guido and Kevin Kleitz for well-timed musical distractions. And last but not least, a special debt of gratitude to Beezo, Big C (a.k.a. the "Wiz") Jimi, Leon, Lil' A, and Farley for incalculable inspiration.

Be a part of the growing GUT HELP™ community!

For the latest news and helpful related products for
The Gut Help™ Program, visit the website at:

www.guthelp.com

For all those who are sick of being sick

INTRODUCTION

Even as I type this, it's still hard to believe the improvement I have made, but the facts can't be denied. Simply put, I've gone from twenty bathroom trips a day to just one or two, and nobody could be more elated about that than me. There is no doubt in my mind that if I did not embark on this journey, I'd still be sick today.

Hoping for a non-surgical solution to relieve my suffering, eight years ago I headed down the road of the unknown, not an easy place to be. I had just gotten out of the hospital, an abscess in my colon had me in agony and emergency surgery was needed. It felt like a wake-up call to take control of my life. After living in denial for twelve years that my ulcerative colitis wasn't making my life more difficult, I finally accepted the fact that it was. Needing the bathroom more than twenty times a day didn't leave room for much else. I couldn't hide it anymore; I couldn't live my life anymore. No more lying. No more excuses for being late to everything. Before I considered drastic surgery, I was going to try a diet that had been known to help others with my condition. Unfortunately for me, it didn't go as planned. The questions seemed to pile up: should I continue with the diet? What could I expect physically, emotionally and spiritually from day to day, or month to month? What was acceptable in the realm of ups and downs? And what about probiotics? Should I take them, and if so, how? What brand should I try and what dosage was best? What should I do when I hit a roadblock? How would I know when it was time to change and try another variable?

Simple… I didn't.

This book evolved out of my long road to freedom. There were many trials both successful and disappointing. I documented all my trials in meticulous journals. After years of only fair results and heart-breaking setbacks, I finally hit upon a unique combination of diet, medication, probiotic supplements, motivation and exercise that would bring my pain and agony to an end.

This is the book that I wish I had when I started caring for my health. It would have saved me years of guessing and frustration. This book is my dream realized; it is meant to inspire you to care about your health and take an active role with your physician in your healing. I am not a doctor and therefore, I cannot give advice, but I have done the next best thing; I'm leaving you a memoir of everything I did and what happened to me physically and spiritually while on the road to recovery. No stone is unturned. I had a lot of tough questions, and I found my answers. Now, I want to share it with you.

The Gut Help™ Program I created was not only a chance for me to heal; it was a fantastic opportunity to improve my life. As optimistic as I am, my resilience was challenged greatly through all my setbacks. Though there were times I wanted to give up, I knew my freedom was worth fighting for. As long as my battle was, I'd walk that road a thousand more times if it meant feeling as good as I do now. If we never tried to change, there would be no personal growth.

I've gone from feeling like my life was a curse and now it's a gift. The bad feelings and negative mindset that used to plague me are disappearing; I never knew this kind of gratefulness. There's so much to see and do - even while I'm healing - and I can't wait to do more of it! It's overwhelming to think that I'd still be trapped where I used to be if I didn't try to find my program. Healing was so worth the effort!

– Journal entry from four months into Trial #13

May your journey be as enlightening as mine, only much shorter. I suffered with this horrific and baffling illness for almost twenty years, I wouldn't want anyone to live with it for twenty seconds. Why waste another minute?

Best wishes for improved health!
Stephen Demirjian

CONTENTS

PART I: A Brief History of Me

1986-1998 Diarrhea and pain and blood, oh my!

C'mon, doesn't that top everyone's wish list? Even before I ever knew what IBD or IBS was, I never liked having to take time out to go the bathroom, let alone spend hours in there. Now that's ironic, or sardonic if you are into laughs, because soon it would be obvious that my body had other plans.

At twenty-one years old I was just wrapping up my junior year at college. Fun, freedom and never even thinking about losing bowel control were luxuries that would soon leave me like M.C. Hammer's fortune. Like all college students, I drank beer, ate poorly, and stayed up late, studying of course!

During midterms in the spring of 1986 I got a bout of diarrhea that just wouldn't go away; it kept me running to the bathroom six to eight times a day. While it was thrilling and made for many romantic conversations, my attitude changed to concerned after a couple of weeks. According to the label, I had reached the end of Pepto Bismol's recommended use range and was now in the highly undesirable "consult your doctor" range. Damn those labels!

Still, I thought it was just a bad stomach bug, so I waited another week to see if the magic pink stuff could get rid of this whatever-it-was from my body. No luck. After three weeks of diarrhea and urgency (a.k.a. "Point me to a bathroom… QUICK!!") it was off to the university doctor for me. I remember he nonchalantly asked if a female resident physician could "sit-in" for my sigmoid scope exam. Oh yeah, that went over big. She never did get to see my hinny show, nor did the test yield any conclusive results. Soon, it was off to a specialist, a *gastroenterologist*. My level of concern that things were not well had now gone from mildly amused to semi-freaked-out.

4

So at the age of twenty-one, while other students were engaging in important activities like playing basketball or making out, I was jolted by the reality of getting my first colonoscopy, which is really just a big word for fun. But I wasn't laughing when the results came back. "Ulcerative colitis?? What's that? What do you mean it's incurable? Ok, so where's the camera crew? This is a joke right?"

Wrong.

I was now a member of a small club that I don't remember applying to. (My doctor explained that approximately 1% of the U.S. population suffered from the illness at that time.) Apparently, the disease had taken up residence in two sections of my large intestine, thus causing all the pain and diarrhea. Right away, the doctor put me on Azulfidine, a popular sulfa-based anti-inflammatory drug for IBD. He said I didn't have to change my diet. So I just kept on eating the way I used to, which was pretty much a well balanced diet of pizza, pizza, and more pizza. And to go with that: Pepsi®, Pepsi®, more Pepsi® and maybe a beer or two. These were my days of getting a salad or two a week. Cooked veggies? What are those? Oh yeah, occasionally. Back then I never doubted that a "Number One" on McDonald's value menu didn't give me all the nutrition I needed. (What's a "Number One"? All us junkies know that's a Big Mac®, fries and a Coke. C'mon!)

So there I was, coming home from the pharmacy with big bottles of pills. I had to take four pills with food, four times a day. I tried to keep my life and activities the same, just with more urgent bathroom trips. As I look back now, I was in denial. Even as I took my pills, it never really hit home that I had a serious illness. I didn't see, or maybe more importantly, I didn't want to see myself as sick. I never told anyone that something was wrong, let alone incurable. I just kept it to myself and hoped that it would magically go away. I still remember thinking each time I'd go to the bathroom that somehow this time it would be normal. I had that thought every day for the next ten years.

Meanwhile, each time I needed the bathroom I hoped it wouldn't be too long so that my roommates wouldn't notice any difference. Oh, the excuses I'd make up! I guess I covered it up pretty well because they never asked me if anything was wrong.

Initially, my condition responded pretty well to the pills, I would only have to go to the bathroom four to six times a day with less cramping and urgency. This was an improvement, but it still wasn't great. My doctor gave me a prescription for Cortisone ("Cort") enemas, which were supposed to keep the inflammation down. These did help ease the pain somewhat on my bad days but not enough for me to overcome my feelings of sheer embarrassment from using them. I could imagine telling my date, "Um, would you excuse me while I go squirt this liquid up my butt and then lie down?" Clearly, the Cort enema era wasn't going to last long for me. But unfortunately, that wasn't going to be the end of them. The "party" was just getting started.

A couple of years passed and I was soon a college grad in the working world. Much to my disappointment, my condition had not cleared up; it had gotten worse. It was 1989 and I needed the bathroom more often, about eight to ten times a day with cramps and increasing pain. Occasionally, I would also have bouts with bleeding and the doctor would then recommend the Cort enemas for a week or two. I was still taking Azulfidine and I was still eating anything I wanted with no diet restrictions. Like most folks, when I wasn't feeling well I ate my favorite comfort foods more often – that's why they call them comfort foods! You know, all that good healthy stuff like cookies, cakes, and soda.

I did the best I could managing my job and personal life while trying not to let the illness control me and my spirit, but the juggling act kept getting tougher. A truly annoying pattern began to develop: now after I'd finish once in the bathroom, I'd almost immediately need to run back and go again. This cycle would repeat itself four to six times and then subside for a few hours. Those hours were precious to get any errands or work done before the next "attack." I'd feel best at those times, happy to be back among the living, to be part of life. But soon I'd get that urgent feeling again, and have to find a bathroom fast. I'd need to go another four to six times and there was very little room for error because in most cases I could not hold off the urgency more than two minutes. That meant I always had to be aware of the nearest bathroom. Always. And to add some game show-like uncertainty, I'd never know if all the stalls would be taken. That was a nightmare! As I began to memorize bathroom locations in all the places I would go, I made mental notes of the ones with many stalls available. I felt trapped in this private torment; it was an awful way to live.

This cycle would repeat again at night. Now it was getting much harder for me to hide my condition but that didn't stop me from trying. I was running out of excuses for my roommates and my nervousness increased around using the bathroom. I began to develop a wall around me. My personality was becoming affected; part of me just went into a shell. I couldn't see any other way. I had to keep going on. Hey, I was a young guy in my prime! As unnatural as the illness seemed, my hiding it seemed completely natural.

I wish I could say that something, some wonder pill or miracle, swooped in and saved me from this daily nightmare of existence. I sure was praying for it. I'd ask my doctors for new treatments constantly. By 1991, I'd moved my residence twice, and had three more doctors, the most prominent gastroenterologists in their respective cities. But the word was always the same, "Nothing new yet." There were inklings in the holistic world, colon cleansing was popular at the time, but that wasn't for folks with IBD or IBS. We were stuck. So I just stayed the course and tried to focus on my work at the time.

I now needed the bathroom ten to fourteen times a day. I developed an allergic reaction to sulfa meds (including Azulfidine) and switched to the popular mesalamine drug, Pentasa® (another form of anti-inflammatory medication). I was now taking Cort enemas and steroids when the bleeding and flare-ups got out of hand, which became several times a year. I was in some kind of stupor, numb really. I put up with all my pain, discomfort, and inconvenience and lived for the few hours when I wasn't on the toilet. I still dreamed about magically healing. I was truly in denial.

I remember sitting in "my office" (a.k.a. the toilet) doing the math in my head saying, "Wow, I've had colitis for five years!" And it wasn't long before I sat there and said, "Wow, I've had colitis for ten years!"

Ten years of this CRAP!

Each year my flare-ups would get longer. In my twelfth year with the illness I was in a flare-up for almost the entire year. Going anywhere from sixteen to twenty plus times a day left me little time for anything else. I should've just installed a cot in the bathroom to make things easier, but you know how small those Boston apartments are.

I couldn't concentrate on any projects or hold a job. I had become agoraphobic (one who's afraid of open or public places), and who wouldn't if they needed the toilet that much? I remember not being able to walk down the driveway to my car without needing to run back in the house for the toilet. Imodium helped somewhat with the urgency issue, but that was really just postponing the inevitable as I would still have to run for the bathroom when the time came.

Bleeding was a daily occurrence without Prednisone (the steroid of choice for IBD). I felt better on the steroids for a little while, but with each round I took, I'd experience even worse side effects. I was at my wit's end, agitated, depressed, exhausted and frustrated by the toll the illness was taking on my loved ones and me. Not only was I in pain, I was wracked with guilt for being grumpy and complaining to them (my only audience) all the time. Amazingly, they never lost their temper with me, even when I certainly did with myself. That's beyond love.

Now, no good story would be complete without the famous line, "Just when you think things couldn't get any worse...." And far be it from me to disappoint you, because that's just what happens here. It's a tough part to write, but as you'll see, sometimes you just got to get down to get up.

It was Mother's Day 1998, and I was begging my girlfriend to take me to the emergency room that morning, as fast as possible! I could barely stand. I had a pain in my "bottom" that was so unbearable I thought I was going to pass out. After twelve years of colitis, you could say that I was familiar with gut and bowel agony, but this was beyond the worst I had ever experienced. I now thought I was going to die from pain after my usual morning diarrhea. So off to the emergency room we went, and thankfully after only an hour wait, a doctor was in to see me.

What followed next is hard to remember because I almost passed out again when he examined me. He didn't know what it was right away, but bless his soul, he immediately got me on morphine and spoke with the surgeon on hand. They needed a specialist and put me in a hospital bed to wait until he got there. It was only a few hours, but even loaded up on as much morphine as I could beg from the nurses, it seemed like an eternity. The pressure and pain was just so unbearable, I couldn't even think about trying to "get comfortable."

Soon, I was into surgery and woke up with some pain but at least no pressure. The doctor said I had suffered from an abscess (an infection) in my colon. Most likely he believed that it came from a cut sustained when inserting one of my prescribed Cortisone enemas. How delightful! As if I needed one more thing to worry about. And with that, they sent me home to heal.

Bowel movements in this post-surgery healing time, as you could imagine, really hurt. The spasmodic like nature of my diarrhea only exacerbated the pain. Having to go so many times a day didn't help either. But with the daily recommended Sitz Baths I began to heal the cut inside and after two weeks the pain from the abscess was gone.

While I was healing from surgery, my dad called one weekend and told me about a book he had found. He said it was about a diet that had helped people with gut troubles like mine. The book, *Breaking the Vicious Cycle*, by Elaine Gottschall, describes how a diet she got from a doctor helped cure her daughter's condition of ulcerative colitis. After her daughter got well, Elaine went on to study the effects of food on the function of the digestive track. Her research and findings are explained in the book.

I remember jumping right to the chapter on the diet and discovering I was going to have to make some significant changes. I was sick of being sick and now willing to do anything to get better. (More on the diet and recipes later, but if you can't wait, jump to Parts 3, 7 and 8.) I knew I was going to be changing all right, but just how I never really expected.

The following chapter encapsulates my eight years of experience with diets, probiotics and medications in the quest to relieve my symptoms.

PART 2: The Trials – A Search for Relief

It all started in May 1998 with a diet and the will to escape from my pain. My father had found the book, *Breaking the Vicious Cycle*, by Elaine Gottschall. Like me, her daughter also suffered with ulcerative colitis, but as a child. She was able to return to health within two years on The Specific Carbohydrate Diet™, a.k.a. the SCD™. Culled from Elaine's years of study, the book presents the science behind the diet that was first pioneered and researched by Drs. Sidney V. and Merrill P. Haas in the early 1950's.

The theory behind the diet was simple: remove the foods that feed the "bad" bacteria in the intestine that contribute to the development of disease. If the bad bacteria's food source is removed, the body can have an opportunity to heal. That basically meant eating no complex carbohydrates like bread, starch, or refined sugars of any kind - no cheeses with lactose and no chocolate either. These foods did not break down into simple sugars that the body could easily digest and thus gave the bad bacteria fuel to thrive and wreak havoc. After reading her book I thought that the logic of the diet seemed promising. And even as a devotee of the junk food lifestyle, I thought, "Why do I want to keep hurting my gut by eating the wrong food? I'll never get better that way! Maybe it's time I started to eat healthy."

It was time to see for myself if the diet worked. Cold turkey was how I chose to start. Elaine's book explained that cheating on the diet would inhibit, if not prevent, any potential healing, so I wasn't interested in doing this half-hearted. I had waited over twelve years to be well and I wanted to get better as fast as possible. Unfortunately, Elaine adds that the diet does not work for everyone, but I was in too much pain not to try it. It didn't seem hard at first, only strange because I had never restricted my foods before. My taste buds might not have been convinced yet, but my gut and my head felt ready to forge ahead.

Upon starting the diet, I immediately had many questions. This was going to be a huge life change, and I wished I had more details on what was going to happen to me, but the details of the road to healing were not included in Elaine's book. And so, the questions seemed to pile up: what could I expect physically, emotionally and spiritually from day to day, or month to month? What was acceptable in the realm of ups and downs? And what about probiotics? Should I take them, and if so, how? What brand should I try and what dosage was best? What should I do when I hit a roadblock? How would I know when it was time to change and try another variable?

Simple… I didn't.

No health professionals could guide me in this course of healing, and at that time, none even believed that diet made a difference. (I had one nutritionist at a prestigious hospital tell me to eat white bread! It was loaded with bad carbs, and therefore, a big SCD™ no-no.) Neither could my physicians counsel me on which probiotics to try nor in what concentrations. I was definitely on my own. Not a comfortable position to be in, but neither was sitting on the toilet all day. For me, I had no choice but to forge ahead and take good notes. It helped that I was a pre-med student with a strong science background and understood research concepts. This did not however, pardon me from being human and suffering from internal and external influences like cravings, depression, bad advice, etc., all of which I have included here because it is relevant information and necessary for an accurate picture as a patient.

At first it may seem hard to believe that I could even make it through thirteen trials over eight years. But isn't that a testament to how awful living with gut illness really is? Taking ownership of my health bore a certain burden no doubt; but if a program could set me free from the horrible pain of a life-long handicap, then I was willing to put in the effort, again and again.

The data that follows is culled directly from my daily journal entries during the eight-year period of research from 1998 to 2006.

SUMMARY OF TRIALS

KEY:

SCD™	= The Specific Carbohydrate Diet™
P	= Pentasa®
OP	= other probiotics
PD	= Primal Defense® probiotics (original formula)
PDNF	= Primal Defense® probiotics (new formula)
N	= Natren® probiotics

TRIAL #1: The Specific Carbohydrate Diet™ (SCD™)

Duration: One year and nine months (May 1998 – January 2000)

Medication taken: Pentasa® (prescribed by my doctor) 1000mg, 3 times/day, Cort enemas (prescribed by my doctor) usually for a two week period or less, Rowasa® enemas (prescribed by my doctor) usually for a two week period or less, and Prednisone (prescribed by my doctor) as needed for cramps, flare-ups and bleeding that wouldn't subside after using the enemas.

Supplements taken: One daily multivitamin, as recommended on the SCD™.

Summary: The SCD™ cut my symptoms in half, but it couldn't do more on it's own.

Trial Highlights:

Within weeks of starting the diet I went from needing the toilet an average of twenty times a day down to an average of twelve. Bloating, pain, cramps and blood had decreased substantially as well as that putrid smell that used to accompany most bowel movements. The feeling was undeniable: my gut was much less burdened while digesting and doing its job. My initial results seemed to support that by removing specific carbohydrates from my diet I was no longer "feeding" the bad bacteria in the intestines, therefore reducing my gut pain and symptoms.

Yet, after four months on the diet it seemed my progress came to a halt. I was going on average eight to ten times a day. Some days I'd have less pain, cramps, diarrhea and spasms while other days would be heavy. Loose, barely formed stools were present almost daily along with post bowel movement pain, which could vary from a little to quite a lot. Blood was still present sporadically (i.e., every couple of weeks).

Sometimes I'd have two good weeks with no cramps, diarrhea and blood, and then I'd have four weeks with. This flare-up pattern continued on for eight months, then a year, then a year and nine months. All the while I kept thinking that what was happening actually had a cause and effect when really there was none. I thought I might just be getting stomach flu or ate something bad, but the amount and pattern of my flare-ups were too frequent to support that idea. I could not see that my healing had come to a stand still. My unwavering belief that healing was just around the corner eventually gave way to the understanding that I was making no furtherprogress.

I wished I had this book then. I had no guide, nothing to compare to. My initial results were promising, but I didn't know what to make of this place I was stuck in. I was frustrated and had nowhere to turn, so I decided to call Elaine herself for an opinion. After describing my experience and results, she said she did not think the diet was working for me. It was very difficult to hear.

I had not yet discovered how to analyze my data by looking at the bigger picture. If I had only stepped back after my progress and looked at my results in just a few subsequent months I would've noticed sooner that the data was similar, and I was not improving. *I learned later, when I found my winning program, that monthly improvement was always evident on some level be it mental focus, energy, stool quality, less bathroom trips, etc.*

Having the illness was bad enough, and knowing this diet healed others but not me just made me feel worse. Like every bad addict, this extremely disheartening news just drove me back to the only thing that made me happy: no food restrictions. Maybe I didn't want to believe that my symptoms were somewhat relieved on the diet. Or maybe, I just forgot how much more pain the diet saved me from. Either way, I was about to find out.

TRIAL #2: No diet restrictions, tried to regulate "bad" carbs

Duration: Five months (February 2000 – June 2000)

Medication taken: Pentasa®, Cort enemas, and Rowasa® enemas.

Supplements taken: Solgar® acidophilus taken as directed on bottle: 2 capsules/ day with meals, each capsule contains 500 million microorganisms (acidophilus was approved by my doctor), Fish oil (1000mg pills, 10/day as recommended by my doctor), and one daily multivitamin.

Summary: The more "bad" carbs (those not on the SCD™) that I ate, the sicker I got.

Trial Highlights:

At first I told myself that I would regulate my "bad" carbs, but that soon gave way to eating all the junk I wanted, anytime. At first, I didn't notice any dramatic changes within days of putting bread and sugar back in my diet. I thought somehow, magically, I could tolerate these SCD™ forbidden foods again. Wrong! Much to my dismay, it took only a week for the putridity, cramps, and diarrhea to increase. What I figured out was that my system had partially cleaned out with the SCD™ and now by eating sugar and bread, I was back to messing it up again. I was back to where I started, needing the toilet approximately twenty times a day.

As my pain increased, my doctor recommended the Cort and Rowasa® enemas. He told me that they've found many patients do best with a regimen of two enemas a week. I took the enemas and felt less discomfort, which fooled me into thinking that progress was being made but it was not. All that was happening was a cycle of hurting my gut with the forbidden foods, then cleansing it with the enemas. I'd use the Cort or Rowasa® enemas for two or three days then discontinue them. I'd eat whatever I wanted and within two days I'd need to go back on the enemas again because the cramps, diarrhea and pain were so heavy. A pattern developed: The more bad carbs I ate, the more I needed the enemas. Soon it felt like I needed one every night!

This started out as a happy time. I felt more like everyone else with no diet restrictions, and that was important to me then. I hadn't really changed my eating habits in my head, so it felt more comfortable to eat with no restrictions like I used to. Slowly I realized my health was getting worse. *While I loved the freedom to eat what I craved, I learned that I was suffering for it.*

I really hated doing the enema procedure. Even though my doctor quoted research that patients did better with the enemas twice weekly, I could not see it as a practical solution for me. Not only were they inconvenient and embarrassing, my pain and discomfort were still present with their use. My quality of life was suffering again.

With the cycle of pain and still unpredictable bathroom needs, this was not adding up as a viable solution for me. I was sick, stressed out, and eating poorly to make myself temporarily feel better. I started to get depressed even before I was about to eat a favorite junk food, because I knew what was going to happen after I ate it. That began to take the enjoyment out of it for me. Out of the pain and results of this trial I was beginning to form a new mindset. I realized I needed to find a better way, but I didn't have it yet. One additional note, I had tried a brand of probiotics during this trial and found no positive or negative effect when taking them according to the recommended dosage, so I discontinued their usage for the next trial.

TRIAL #3: Dairy free diet

Duration: Two months (July 2000-August 2000)

Medication taken: Pentasa®, Cort enemas, and Rowasa® enemas.

Supplements taken: Fish oil, and one daily multivitamin.

Summary: My symptoms are not caused by just dairy.

Trial Highlights:

Upon mentioning my gut pain to a close friend, it came out in the conversation that he too had gut trouble. His condition was called Spastic Colon, and he kept his flare-ups to an absolute minimum (i.e., once or twice a year) with a dairy free diet. He said his health was great, he had no social restrictions and was able to live a "normal" life as long as he stayed away from dairy products. So I decided to try his diet too, to think it could work for me. I never considered that it could be just dairy causing all the trouble. (Although, in 1994 I was found to be lactose intolerant after a gastroenterologist tested me.)

I continued to eat whatever I wanted (including bread and sugar), but I stayed away from just dairy products. I began having rice or soymilk in the morning with whole grain cereals. My symptoms did not improve. I also needed the enemas again, just as in Trials #1 and #2. All my familiar symptoms (pain, cramps, diarrhea, multiple bathroom trips, and occasional blood) were still present, as well as my old fears about urgency and leaving the house.

Again, this started as a happy time because I thought I had my problem figured out. Actually, I really just wanted to believe this new approach was working when it really wasn't. When I experienced the heavy physical pain again, I couldn't deny the facts: this trial didn't work either. Obviously, I had proved that dairy was not the only thing that made my symptoms worse.

I was sitting on the sidelines again and I hated it. I was now more sad and desperate than I was in the previous trials and it felt like the drama of my battle was increasing, challenging me. Why couldn't this simple solution work for me too? How much harder did I have to try to help myself? I wished I could wake up from this nightmare like in the movies. But unfortunately, everyday upon awakening I realized I was still sick and in a lot of physical pain. I remained at the point where I couldn't even make it out of the house.

Confused and frustrated, this was another blow to my spirits when this trial failed. But after a brief period of feeling sorry for myself, I realized I had to try again. I called a physician who practiced holistic medicine; Elaine recommended him.

TRIAL #4: No Dairy, Bread or Potatoes diet

Duration: One year and seven months (September 2000 – March 2002)

Medication taken: Pentasa®, Cort enemas, Rowasa® enemas, Prednisone, and Prilosec®.

Supplements taken: Kyo-Dophilus® 2 pills/day with meals as recommended on label. (This was another popular brand of probiotics I decided to try; each pill contained 1.5 billion live microorganisms.) L-Glutamine (a muscle building amino acid as directed by the holistic doctor, 1000mg/day), Fish oil, and one daily multivitamin.

Summary: Even though the holistic doctor removed some resistant starches, this trial proved they're all bad to a sick gut.

Trial Highlights:

The holistic doctor recommended that I try removing bread and potatoes as well as dairy from my diet reasoning that these were complex carbohydrate rich, that is, harder carbs to digest for some people with gut illness. This regimen seemed like the SCD™ but allowed me to have corn, soy, rice and sugar, which of course, I indulged in. That made life a little easier convenience-wise (rice cereals, rice bread, soy milk etc.) but as my journal showed, a day or two after I ate these foods I would get that putrid smell during bathroom trips; my signal that these foods were fermenting in my colon and not being digested.

Some days I'd have more blood, other days more diarrhea and more bathroom trips. But on almost everyday my least favorite of all symptoms, urgency, was present and I would have several painful bouts of cramps. These symptoms were definitely worse than when I was on just the SCD™ alone. During this time I had two extended flare-ups that lasted approximately six months each. I was put on Prednisone for extended periods during this trial and I was using the Cort and Rowasa® almost weekly. I had tried another brand of probiotics (Kyo-Dophilus®) during this trial and found no positive benefit when taking it according to the recommended dosage. I also developed acid reflux during this trial and was treated with Prilosec® by my doctor. This condition disappeared in Trial #5 6-13 and medication was no longer needed.

I was on this program for far too long because of denial that the previous Trial #1 (with the SCD™) did help somewhat. The high I got from forbidden foods was also no match for my level of discipline at the time, but a realization was going to help change that. Finally, I began to see that when I ate whatever I wanted, I needed more drugs. And for me, they just didn't manage the subsequent pain enough.

The bottom line was, I was still in pain and needed the bathroom way too much during the day. This trial showed me that I can do a lot more to manage my pain by not feeding the bad bacteria in my large intestine with starchy and sugary foods of any kind. Being on the SCD™ was better than being off it, but now I was still stuck somewhere in the middle.

TRIAL #5: Primal Defense®

Duration: Three months (April 2002 – June 2002)

Medication taken: Pentasa® and Prilosec®.

Supplements taken: Primal Defense®, Perfect Food®, FYI®, and Omega-Zyme® - all manufactured by Garden of Life™, and one daily multivitamin.

Summary: There was no magic pill that would make my stomach tolerate sugary or starchy foods no matter how much I wished it were true. My body was better on the SCD™.

Trial Highlights:

After reviewing my options I decided to try a new probiotic, Primal Defense®, manufactured by Garden of Life™. I followed their recommended diet that focused on a reduction of sugar and wheat. Primal Defense® is a different type of probiotic from the others I had tried; it is made using Homeostatic™ Soil Organisms (HSO™), which are basically bacteria from the soil. I bought a bottle of the pills and followed the directions for advance use, which was recommended for people with intestinal illness according to their literature.

Garden of Life™ recommended increasing by one pill a week for advanced use until a maximum dosage of twelve pills is reached. It went on to say that the person should stay at the max dose for three months, then gradually reduce to a maintenance dose of three per day for life. So that was my plan. I started, as the directions recommended, with one pill on an empty stomach, twenty to thirty minutes before a meal and increased by one pill a week. As the weeks went on, I spread out the pills before breakfast, lunch and dinner. Early results looked promising.

In the literature I received about Primal Defense®, it mentioned other Garden of Life™ products to try, namely: Perfect Food® (a super green vitamin supplement), FYI®

(a natural supplement "For Your Inflammation"), and Omega-Zyme® (additional digestive enzymes to help breakdown carbohydrate rich foods like cake, etc.). According to their literature, all of these products seemed to promise that they could relieve my symptoms. They were marketed specifically for gut ailments like mine. I figured I had nothing to lose so I decided to try all three according to their directions soon after I started Primal Defense®.

My journal notes show that while Perfect Food® increased my energy, I was also having more of my symptoms because it contained many ingredients that were forbidden on the SCD™. With FYI® I did not notice any significant benefit in inflammation reduction as advertised. To me, the Omega-Zyme® marketing (pictures of cookies and cakes with the slogan "enjoy your favorite foods") sent the mixed message that eating cakes and cookies were OK so long as I took the pills. Unfortunately, this was not the case, as my symptoms of bloating, gas, painful cramps and diarrhea all increased. I noticed that as I increased the breads and sugars I ate - even with the Omega-Zyme® - my adverse reactions also increased.

My holistic doctor suggested that Omega-Zyme® may be "over-digesting" my food. He recommended that I stop all other supplements and lower my Primal Defense® to the amount I was taking before cramping (i.e., nine pills) and see if that helped. It decreased my painful symptoms within four days.

Unfortunately, Omega-Zyme®'s marketing message was giving me license to eat the very foods that Primal Defense® said to stay away from. My results showed an increase in pain and symptoms, making it difficult, if not impossible, for me to heal. I realized I had gotten caught up in the promise of a "magic pill." I was beginning to understand that there was no magic pill that would make my stomach tolerate sugary or starchy foods no matter how much I wished it were true. Finally, it was perfectly clear that my body was better on the SCD™ and that doing it halfway was not only more difficult, it just didn't work. I wanted to get back to the SCD™ immediately, but this time I was going to take comfort in the diet's restrictions. I wrote a new favorite motto in my journal:

The diet of "no" is much easier than the diet of "maybe."

TRIAL #6: SCD™ and Primal Defense®

Duration: Seven months (July 2002 – January 2003)

Medication taken: Pentasa®.

Supplements taken: Primal Defense®, L-Glutamine, and one daily multivitamin.

Summary: Just because the SCD™ lists a food as OK, it does not necessarily mean that it's OK for you.

Trial Highlights:

As I dug in and began the SCD™ with strict adherence, I was continuing to experience intense bloating and cramps. It was perplexing. What was causing this reaction? I would've expected to be moving right along in my progress, instead, I still needed the bathroom quite often, averaging over thirteen times a day. The pain, often so heavy it would almost knock me out, led me to believe something was definitely not working. I immediately began to lower my Primal Defense® intake since that seemed to help at the end of my last trial.

As I decreased my pills, my symptoms still did not seem to improve, so I continued to decrease by two pills a week until I was down to zero by the end of November. Was my earlier success with Primal Defense® a fluke? Was it causing more problems? I was following the diet fanatically. It was all I could guess.

I called my holistic doctor and he asked if I had been eating peanuts. He reminded me that peanuts have a large amount of lactose in them and I, like most IBD and IBS patients, am lactose intolerant. It was true; restarting the diet was challenging for me and I had been eating peanut butter as a snack, three or four times each day. I remembered that the SCD™ recommends staying away from peanuts until six months into the diet, which I did the first time I tried the SCD™ and only ate them thereafter on a very limited basis. But being lactose intolerant, I may have to stay away from them altogether; so I buckled down, and crossed peanuts and peanut butter off my list for the time being.

Slowly, the painful bloating and excessive cramping subsided. I was back to needing the bathroom approximately ten times a day like I was on just the SCD™ in Trial #1. I had stopped taking Primal Defense® by December 2002, and unfortunately, I stayed in this difficult place of pain and repeated flare-ups hoping things would improve on just the diet for another month. They didn't. Because my spirit and focus were so affected by the pain of this trial I had not fully realized that it was the peanut butter that was halting my progress and not the Primal Defense® as I had guessed. While cooking one day, I came across a bottle of Primal Defense® in my cupboard and decided to try it again.

It's important to note that just because the SCD™ lists a food as OK, it does not necessarily mean that it's OK for you. This lesson of not paying attention to my food journal more often was a costly one. It took me months to figure it out, but staying away from peanuts was better for me even though it was a favorite. To me, being in less pain was better than any peanuts or peanut butter ever tasted. I was back on track and determined not to let this further restriction stop me.

I suffered greatly during this period wishing I had a book like this one to help me get some kind of understanding for interpreting results. Restricting my diet even further, trying to be my own doctor, and not improving made this one of my most challenging times. Originally, I was crushed to have to remove peanut butter from my diet. It was such a convenient, tasty snack and outstanding energy source that losing it was a huge blow to my happiness at first. But from this low-point of pain and frustration came answers and hope; I began to develop a deeper understanding of the affect of chronic illness and diet restrictions. These observations fueled my spirit, and I started formulating many of the successful methods I used to overcome roadblocks, which are included later on in this book.

TRIAL #7: SCD™ and Primal Defense®, No Peanuts

Duration: One year (February 2003 – January 2004)

Medication taken: Pentasa®, Cort enemas, and Canasa® suppositories (as prescribed by doctor).

Supplements taken: Primal Defense®, and one daily multivitamin.

Summary: Dramatic healing occurs.

Trial Highlights:

To say I was fanatical about staying on the diet this time would be right on. I was glad to be back on it. And with the tips I developed for myself (see Part 4) it was now easy to stay on it. I was so committed to the diet that I'd be hesitant to take even a Tylenol®, or any over-the-counter meds, for concern that their inactive ingredients could be non-diet safe (most over-the-counter pills have starches as fillers).

For the times I would need over-the-counter pain relief, I would have my "Tylenol®" (acetaminophen) made with no fillers by a compounding pharmacist. If I had to take an over-the-counter medicine then I would, but I always looked at the labels and tried to choose the one with the least amount of diet infractions. I stayed away from all aspirin and ibuprofen products like Advil® because like many people, they irritated my stomach and caused bleeding.

With peanuts out of the picture, a commitment to my program of the SCD™ with Primal Defense® paid off instantly. In my first week alone, bathroom visits were cut almost in half (down to about six per day) and my energy increased, energy that I forgot I ever had. That was an incredible feeling. These improvements were monumental not just because I was feeling better, but as a result of fewer bathroom trips, I was getting more time back in my day. Life was beginning to turn around, and I was rightfully excited.

My journal entries show an important pattern developing for me by the third pill of Primal Defense®: almost always on the third day of each pill increase I would get a little more of my symptoms. At first it felt like an old flare-up, but it was almost always over in a day or two and occasionally included bleeding. This did not fit the M.O. of an old flare-up that usually lasted weeks or months and often included frequent bleeding. The Primal Defense® literature called this a "Herxheimer reaction," a short-term immunological reaction to treatment in which the body experiences an increase in previous symptoms. Sometimes I would experience brief headache or flu-like symptoms. It was nothing severe. For me, it was usually slightly increased cramping, looser stools and a few more bathroom visits. This increase in symptoms almost always calmed back down within two days. I'd then enjoy the last two days of the week with a stronger gut feeling and increased overall energy that got me ready for the next pill increase. This pattern lasted all the way until I reached the max dosage of twelve pills. These Herxheimer reactions seemed to be a necessary passage to better health.

Occasionally, certain pill increases were more challenging (i.e., more pain, cramps or diarrhea) and I'd need a few more days to get comfortable again. On those weeks that I didn't bounce back in two days, I'd wait another week for the next pill increase, giving my body more time to adjust. It made the transitions smoother. I never physically needed more than two weeks to adjust. My notes show that I was actually enjoying the process of each new pill increase. It was exciting to move forward on the weeks that I could. It gave me an overwhelming feeling of accomplishment as I was usually rewarded with newfound wellness, be it improved concentration, more energy, or improved bathroom trips.

By the fourth pill, stools began to improve and become more formed. A quote from my journal during this week read, *"I'm excited about going out and not the least bit worried if I'll need the toilet. If I ever did, I'd now have plenty of time to get there, and that's without Imodium! I know I'm getting better because my mind is on the time I'm having, not my body."*

At five pills (seven weeks) I needed the bathroom about three or four times a day (aside from the weekly Herxheimer reaction days were I'd go approximately four to six times a day). Usually my first bathroom trip of the day took the longest, sometimes up to twenty minutes. But at least the others were faster, and that was an improvement. I actually felt well enough to hold down a job again and that felt like a milestone.

At this time, I often experienced colonic soreness (occasionally strong) after using the bathroom, but I could usually attribute that to eating too many raw nuts or raw veggies the day or days before. Some days if soreness was heavy, I had good results from taking some acetaminophen and using a Canasa® (mesalamine) suppository that was prescribed by my doctor. I also tried to go easy on the nuts or raw veggies the next few days.

While on my sixth pill (eight weeks), I caught a bad stomach flu that necessitated cutting back to three pills. After the flu passed, I worked my way back up from three to eight pills by the end of my third month with only a few minor challenges along the way. By my fourth month, I was up to nine pills.

"Moving up to nine pills was very challenging," my journal states, "…symptoms were a bit stronger, very similar to the challenge of five pills." This increase needed two weeks for me to feel strong enough to move forward again. Even though the increase in symptoms tapered by the end of the first week, I decided to stay on another week and enjoy my new level of health during my brother's wedding celebration in NYC the following weekend. My progress wasn't showing so much in the bathroom yet, but there was no mistaking a strong feeling of overall well-being and body confidence. I decided to test my newfound freedom by setting a personal record of seeing four different rock concerts that weekend. I never did that even before I got sick.

While at ten pills I went through a stressful period of divorce, and selling our home, and moving. My notes show that I did have a flare-up and used Cort enemas to calm it down until the move was over. During this month I just held on at ten Primal Defense® pills, I didn't want to challenge my gut until the flare calmed down.

Once the move was over, I was getting more sleep and beginning to adjust to my new life. I was ready to increase my Primal Defense® dosage. On August 17, 2003, approximately six and a half months since I began this trial, I was at eleven pills. My notes show that this pill increase was taken well, with no challenging symptoms to report.

In a week I was at the top dose recommended by the manufacturer (twelve pills a day). I felt happy and accomplished; it took me just under seven months to make it to the "top." Now needing the bathroom two or three times a day, stools were formed well, but not perfect yet. I was still having occasional spasms and blood in stools; the only other symptom I had lingering was my post movement soreness. For this, I was taking my prescribed Canasa® suppositories twice a day, and that was helping to soothe the lower section of the rectum.

In two weeks I was scheduled to have a colonoscopy; the last one I had was a year and half earlier, and the results were not good (February 28, 2002, while not on the SCD™ or Primal Defense®). The report from that colonoscopy showed I had much inflammation in the colon. There was active colitis in my transverse and descending colon as well as the rectum.

As of September 17, 2003, I had been on Primal Defense® and the SCD™ for seven months. I was using Canasa® suppositories twice a day and taking my Pentasa® as directed, 1000 mg three times a day. I just knew I was going to be in for a good report because I felt much better in my guts, especially the mid section and descending colon areas on the left side of my body; still, I wanted to hear that the colon was healing from my doctor. Probably, that made me one of the first people ever to look forward to having a colonoscopy.

After the procedure, one of my doctors came in to talk with me as I was in the recovery room. I remember him looking a bit stunned. I didn't know if he had good news or bad, then he smiled. It was tremendous to hear him say, "Everything looks great, so keep up with the diet and whatever you're doing." This was a very happy day.

He called again in a few days and informed me that the biopsies from the exam were very good. He said I only had active colitis now in just the last four inches of the rectum. In the previous scope, the cecum (the start of the large intestine) and the ascending colon were the only normal cells; all else were active colitis. This year the biopsies showed that the cecum and the ascending colon were still normal cells but the rest were inactive colitis cells to the last four inches of the rectum. This was fantastic news! In just seven months on the SCD™ and Primal Defense® together with Pentasa®, we had a strong indication I was healing the areas of the illness.

After the colonoscopy, I stayed at twelve pills for the remainder of the recommended three-month period. Thankfully, the prep procedure of drinking the Phospho-Soda to flush the intestine did not wipe out the progress I had made. My journal shows that I continued going to the bathroom at a rate of two or three times a day during this period. The second time was most often within an hour of the first in the morning. I continued with Canasa® suppositories twice a day to help relieve post soreness. By the end of the three-month period my post soreness was gone and I no longer needed them. My journal read,

"Gut feels so much better - no need for Canasa anymore - haven't even thought about it. That nagging soreness in my rectum after using the bathroom is finally gone! Neither do I think about the bathroom when I'm out. It's just incredible! This is a real big milestone of a step; they all are for that matter. Each new one brings some new freedom; I feel like I'm getting put back together again! I just can't completely describe how overwhelming that feels: to be finally escaping this condition that's kept me down for so long."

As recommended, at the end of three months on twelve pills per day I then gradually lessened my dosage of Primal Defense® by two pills per week to get down to the maintenance dose of three pills a day. I didn't record any significant changes until after the second month back down at three pills. That's when improvements really became very noticeable. The volume of smaller stools was transforming to fewer, and bigger normal sized stools. Going to the bathroom now felt much like it used to before I got ulcerative colitis. And just as amazing, a bathroom visit now could be completed in a once unthinkable time of less than five minutes! I now needed the bathroom only once, or at most, twice a day. I had no urgency. No cramping. No pain during or after. No spasms and, of course, no diarrhea. I would even get a charge of energy after using the bathroom like I used to, a "normal" feeling I had long forgotten. I felt like I was back to life and it felt better than I ever imagined. A favorite comment from my journal at this time read, "It's amazing all the things you can do when you're not on the toilet!" Oh yes, how true it is.

My journal notes of bathroom visits and symptoms during this period were again invaluable. Once I got the hang of seeing the pattern of my Herxheimer reactions, I was able to plan my pill increases according to my work/life schedule. For example, if I was going to be traveling on the third or fourth day of a pill increase and it wouldn't be convenient to deal with the expected increase in symptoms, then I'd hold off on that pill increase until I was back home for a week. So some pill dosages I'd stay at for a week, and others, occasionally two or three.

The key was that I balanced listening to my body with my life and work demands, not forgetting that the goal was to keep moving forward. It was almost like a video game. Move forward but don't push it was my motto. I found much success in keeping my pace slow and steady. By doing so, at the end of the third month, I felt ready to begin some light exercise with walking. Again, I did whatever I could handle, never pushing it. It felt good to just want to exercise again. It was wonderful to be outside in spring, my healing seemed perfectly timed with the season. I was grateful!

Clearly, this trial was marked with much happiness and great feelings of personal triumph. But unfortunately, in my twelfth month, I started to feel so good being almost completely healed that I lost sight of what got me there. I started to complain about the inconvenience of always having to take Primal Defense® on an empty stomach and began to think about getting a less expensive probiotic. I was well now, right? In late January 2004, I stopped taking Primal Defense® and replaced it with another probiotic.

If only I had reviewed my notes from a year before, I might have thought otherwise. Unfortunately, after all these great strides forward, I would let my recovery go to my head, and forget that golden rule: *if it ain't broke, don't fix it!* I would soon mess with my successful program and suffer needlessly to re-learn this important lesson.

TRIAL #8: SCD™ and other probiotics

Duration: Four months (February 2004 – May 2004)

Medication taken: Pentasa®, Cort enemas, Rowasa® enemas, Prednisone, and Canasa® Suppositories.

Supplements taken: Acidophilus Pearls™ (one daily with food as recommended on label) each pill contains 1 billion live microorganisms, Lyo-San® Acidophilus (up to three daily with food as recommended on label) each pill contains 3 billion Yogurt/acidophilus live microorganisms, and one daily multivitamin.

Summary: Don't mess with success! Not all probiotics yield results. I don't experience flare-ups when my probiotics are successful.

Trial Highlights:

Within weeks of removing Primal Defense® and switching to a new probiotic, Acidophilus Pearls™, all of my old symptoms were coming back. And because they came back slowly, it made me think that anything but the change in probiotics was responsible. "Oh it must be the water," I'd say or, "I must have gotten food poisoned." But after a month without Primal Defense®, I was having flare-ups again. Just when I thought I was back to my old self, the nightmare of my illness returned. All my old symptoms were back and I was miserable!

By two months on the new Pearls™ probiotic, I was back to needing the bathroom over ten times a day. I was stuck again with all the symptoms I wanted to forget: horrible pain and cramps, bleeding and diarrhea, and those awful rapid-fire multiple bathroom trips. When the bleeding showed up, I notified my doctor and he put me on a heavy dose of Prednisone. As if I wasn't depressed about my condition already, within a week the Prednisone was making me even more irritable, topped off with what felt like an evil, non-stop caffeine buzz. I also needed Cort enemas as well, and I was still having flare-up-like symptoms. After three months of this, I spoke to a friend who had good results from eating yogurt made with no starch or sugar (see Part 8, Favorite Recipes) and an acidophilus supplement called Lyo-san®. I decided to try both as well, and I discontinued the Pearls™.

Another month went by. No positive changes. I blamed every piece of food I was eating. You would've thought that I was getting food poisoned at every meal. This was obviously untrue. I was eating the same good, healthy SCD™ foods I had prepared for many years. I trudged on thinking that the diet would pull me out of this. It did not. After four months of suffering painful flare-ups, exhaustion, and frustration, I finally decided to carefully review my journal entries for a possible cause. I discovered that it was shortly after getting off Primal Defense® that all my troubles started. It was the only change.

This four-month period in flare-ups bore an important discovery in my fight for recovery: flare-ups are confusing!! They can make you feel like you did something wrong, or ate something that wasn't SCD™ approved, even if you are strictly following the diet as I was. Even worse, the sheer pain of a flare-up is enough to cloud anybody's good judgment. Add that to any commitments and pressure you might be feeling in a normal day, and suddenly just trying to help yourself becomes a lesson in frustration. Many things can trigger a flare-up: a new food allergy, a colonoscopy, a change in diet, food poisoning, or simply the illness itself. This trial showed me that I don't experience flare-ups when my probiotics are successful.

That's why it's important that I stayed on the diet so strictly; it made tracking the change in symptoms much easier. But the key was tracking. It won't do any good to make notes in my journals if I don't review them at least weekly. I would have been able to save myself months of pain and depression if I did so, and maybe I could've saved my progress. I had gotten so used to feeling good that by the end of the last trial I wasn't in the habit of checking my journal notes after I wrote them anymore. Remember, at the time I was actually complaining that I had to take the probiotics before every meal. Well, that's human nature; the rush of finally enjoying my life again was such a thrill that it blinded my better judgment.

When I finally reviewed my journals, the only difference was obvious: the change in the probiotic. All I had to do was look back to the time before the last trial when I started Primal Defense® and compare my present symptoms; they were exactly the same. Then I read what happened as I started the Primal Defense® and it was right there in my notes - I was healing! My symptoms were decreasing; it was completely obvious. The good news is that at least I figured it out in only four months.

For the future, the fact that I started to have so many flare-ups should've been the first signal that something had changed with my method. It's true; some flare-ups are expected in the beginning, they are simply the nature of this illness. But since I found they decrease as the healing occurs, that should've been my tip-off that something in my trial had changed. This trial also pointed out the many important variables involved, such as the nature of intestinal bacteria, and the specific strains and concentrations of probiotics.

TRIAL #9: SCD™, Primal Defense®, and Pentasa®

Duration: Three months (June 2004 – August 2004)

Medication taken: Pentasa®, and Rowasa® enemas.

Supplements taken: Primal Defense®, and one daily multivitamin.

Summary: Certain probiotics contain the right strains for progress.

Trial Highlights:

I started this trial hoping that I could jump right back in where I left off with Primal Defense® four months previous. But when I tried starting back with three pills a day, the pain, heavy cramps, and diarrhea increased; I was detoxing too quickly. My progress from the year previous was lost, and I had to start at the beginning dose of one pill a day. Of course this was disheartening, but I was happy at least to see the progress again. Within four days of being back at the one pill dosage, I no longer needed the Rowasa® enemas I was taking at night.

This time I could increase my dosage of Primal Defense® much faster. Each week I was able to move up to the next pill dosage with only light detoxing symptoms. This was a big difference from my body's initial reaction to the pill increases the year before. Within three months, I was at the top dosage, twelve pills per day. My health was improving again.

In the previous trial, I was fighting off the horrible feelings of the illness and losing my progress. In this trial, while getting better on Primal Defense® again, I had to fight the feelings of extreme sadness and remorse for getting off it to begin with. But it balanced out with just being grateful for making forward progress. I was hoping I could repeat the same success from last year. All I had to do was stay the course, and do just what I did last year. Which sounds much easier than it actually was. In reality, I was very anxious to get back to that glorious state of wellness I once knew. I wanted to be well again more than anything.

Pulling out of my horrible down turn in symptoms within the first week back on Primal Defense® made an important point: certain probiotics contain the right strains for progress. Without them, I stayed locked in a holding pattern of constant flare-ups and symptoms.

TRIAL #10: SCD™, Primal Defense®, NO Pentasa®

Duration: Three months (September 2004 – November 2004)

Medication taken: None.

Supplements taken: Primal Defense®, and one daily multivitamin.

Summary: Without Pentasa®, my forward progress stops.

Trial Highlights:

So you'd think I'd leave well enough alone, right? Wrong! Now I had begun to question whether my medication, Pentasa®, was doing anything to help my cause. There is so much discussion about overmedicating and since I was feeling so well, I began to question the need for my medication. My doctor had prescribed Pentasa® for me as a non-steroid, anti-inflammatory drug and I was soon going to learn (the hard way of course) that it actually was helping. So I took Pentasa® out of my program. By mid-September 2004, without my doctor's knowledge, I had weaned off Pentasa® from twelve pills a day, to none. A great test for science, but not for me, as it would prolong my recovery yet again.

This trial showed a slow decline in my stools until they were small and thin. I had increased inflammation, more bleeding, gut tightening, cramps and spasms. Urgency also increased for me during this trial, and I hate urgency. Like Trial #8, this slow decline made it more difficult to trace the change back to the removal of the Pentasa®. The nature of gut pain made me always want to blame something immediate rather than suspect it was a change from weeks before. Again, I thought it was something new that was the culprit.

In October 2004, one month into hitting the max dose of twelve Primal Defense® pills, I was confused and frustrated at what could be causing my decline so I phoned a distributor of the Primal Defense® product. I didn't tell them I stopped taking my

Pentasa® because I didn't realize the drug played an important role yet. They believed that I had "maxed out" on Primal Defense® and I needed to come back down in my dosage.

I did not experience these symptoms in my successful Trial #7, but I was also on Pentasa® at that time as well. I hadn't put it together yet, so I was a bit bewildered. Feeling awful, I followed their recommendation and dropped back down to three pills. I stayed there for two months as they directed and looked for improvement. While some pain lessened, all my symptoms were still present, especially inflammation. I was going about six to eight times a day and the quality of stools wasn't good. I was worse now then during my successful Trial #7 at the same dosage of Primal Defense®.

In November 2004, I began to suspect that it was the Pentasa® that had helped keep my inflammation down during the healing on Primal Defense® and the SCD™. Because of my good notes, I was able to trace back and figure out that it was the only variable I had changed, but this time, I figured it out much quicker. My suspicion was correct, as my symptoms began to improve within days of getting back on the Pentasa®.

I was elated to quickly discover that Pentasa® was actually helping my healing efforts. This was yet another important trial. It proved that without Pentasa®, my forward progress was stopped.

TRIAL #11: SCD™, Primal Defense®, and Pentasa®

Duration: Four months (December 2004 – March 2005)

Medication taken: Pentasa®.

Supplements taken: Primal Defense®, and one daily multivitamin.

Summary: Progress is made rapidly with the right elements in place until the threat of reformulated probiotics.

Trial Highlights:

Within a couple days of getting back on Pentasa® at my old dose (1000mg/3 times/day) my flared symptoms started to ease. The bleeding and irritation subsided, and my stools were better formed. Here, as in Trial #10, I was a little too anxious to get back to feeling good. I was able to increase my Primal Defense® one per week with little discomfort up until my tenth pill. At that time I was averaging about two to four bathroom trips a day, but I was very uncomfortable. It seems I had gone up too fast in my Primal Defense®, and I was now suffering with increasing cramps and bloating throughout the day. I decided to back off on my dosage, and I didn't get comfortable until I was down to seven Primal Defense® pills a day. In a couple of weeks I worked my way back up to nine pills a day. Everything seemed OK, the cramps and bloating subsided as expected.

This trial undoubtedly showed the positive effects of Pentasa® on my system. For me, it was clear that Pentasa® was effective in reducing inflammation so that the SCD™ and Primal Defense® could help me heal. With the immediate improvement in stool quality and reduction of urgency and cramps, there was no denying the powerful roll Pentasa® plays in my body. It was definitely helping my cause, a much needed player on my winning team.

I knew my program was solid. I was now at nine pills and experiencing the same progress I had once before. I proved that not only could my success be repeated but also how important each piece of the puzzle was to the healing process. Without Pentasa®, my stomach was too inflamed for healing to take place. Without the SCD™, there were too many undigested carbohydrates in my intestines that fed the bad bacteria. And finally, without Primal Defense®, I could not progress in healing.

I placed a call to my Primal Defense® distributor to share my recent results and place a new order. During the call, it came out that Primal Defense® had been reformulated! They were no longer manufacturing the original formula I had been using with success; I couldn't buy it anywhere. My questions came fast and furious, "When was anybody going to make an announcement? Why would they reformulate this product now?" Let alone that I was counting on this supplement and had just taken seven years to prove I couldn't heal without it. I had only a few bottles left of the original formula; what was going to happen to my progress now?

TRIAL #12: SCD™, Primal Defense® (new formula) & Pentasa®

Duration: Two months (April 2005 – May 2005)

Medication taken: Pentasa®.

Supplements taken: Primal Defense® (new formula) and one daily multivitamin.

Summary: Changing probiotic strains stops forward progress.

Trial Highlights:

I called Garden of Life™ customer service in an effort to get some answers about the reformulation of Primal Defense®. The rep told me that some probiotic strains were taken out and others were put in, but I was never satisfied with the explanations why. The worst news was that the two formulas were not interchangeable; I would have to start again from scratch and lose my progress. I couldn't help but wonder why they'd change the formula if the product was working.

The Garden of Life™ rep referred me to a few professionals that used the product; I was able to reach one of them, a chiropractor that helped formulate the pill. He gave me some suggestions, and I developed a plan to wean down on the old formula and build up the new formula based on those suggestions. I was at a dosage of seven old formula pills a day, and I would now swap out an old formula pill for a new formula pill each week until I was at seven new formula pills. I'd then continue to add new formula pills until I reached my old max dose of twelve pills.

That was the plan.

But I never made it. My initial results told me right away that there was a big difference between the two formulas. My guts were cramping severely, my stool quality was poor, and diarrhea was frequent. I didn't give up though; I continued for two more weeks until I got up to three new formula pills a day and the pain was so bad all week that I couldn't go on. After speaking with the chiropractor again, I tried to take out all the new formula for a week and then try to increase it more slowly. That didn't work either. I was passing lots of mucus and having such extreme spasms, blood, cramps and overall pain, that it was too much to continue. It was obvious that it wasn't working. This trial was over for me. I could not repeat my successful results with the new formula of Primal Defense®. I stopped taking it and stayed at four pills of the old formula.

My healing had come to halt and I was devastated. And after I had finally found something that worked too! I actually wondered if I ever would again, now with no old formula of Primal Defense® being manufactured, my health was back in jeopardy. "Well kid," a science teacher once told me, "them's the breaks!" Yes, the breaks indeed.

I began searching the Internet to find other probiotic supplements. I found a company with probiotics that looked hopeful. I got a break, and this time, it was a good one.

TRIAL #13: SCD™, Natren® Probiotics, and Pentasa®

Duration: June 2005 – present

Medication taken: Pentasa®.

Supplements taken: Natren® Megadophilus® dairy free powder, Natren® Bifido Factor® dairy free powder, my own yogurt with Natren® Yogurt Starter (rich in Lactobacillus bulgaricus – see Part 8, Favorite Recipes), and one daily multivitamin. Eventually, I worked up to using the Natren® 3-in-1 Healthy Trinity® capsules that contain all three strains.

Summary: With careful research, I found a supplement that worked.

Trial Highlights:

The probiotic manufacturer I found was called Natren®. I researched their website and learned as much as I could about their company. They have been a producer of quality probiotics for over twenty-five years. I liked their product line; it was simple and straightforward. Natren® Healthy Trinity® contained only three probiotic strains, not fourteen like Primal Defense®. Each of the three strains was chosen because they are the predominant strains in a healthy intestinal tract: namely, Lactobacillus acidophilus (predominant in the small intestine), Bifidobacterium bifidum (predominant in the large intestine), and Lactobacillus bulgaricus that functions throughout the intestines. There are many varieties of these strains, but through much research, Natren® selected three specific types of these strains that were most effective at promoting a healthy intestinal flora and chasing away harmful bacteria.

Natren® suggests using all three probiotic products together because they work in conjunction, hence the name Healthy Trinity®. I wanted to start out with the single Healthy Trinity® 3-in-1 capsule, but a Natren® rep explained that it was a very high concentration and best worked up to. Being that I had experience with probiotics before, I took that advice. Because I'm lactose intolerant, I ordered the dairy free powder version of the Megadophilus® and Bifido Factor®. I used my homemade yogurt (see Part 8, Favorite Recipes) with Natren® Yogurt Starter as my source of the Lactobacillus bulgaricus strain. My diet and lactose intolerance prevented me from using Natren® Digesta-Lac® capsules as the L. bulgaricus source.

Like Primal Defense®, I took the Natren® probiotic powders twenty minutes before a meal. I started with the recommended one half teaspoon of each per day mixed into an eight ounce glass of unchilled spring water. I made a simple schedule that was easy to remember: take my Megadophilus® in the morning before breakfast and my Bifido Factor® before my last snack. This worked well, as I occasionally found the bifidum made me a little sleepy.

By end of the second week, I was down to reliably having three to six movements a day, depending on the Herxheimer reactions. These results came a little sooner than they did on my successful Primal Defense® Trial #7; I was excited to be heading in a positive direction. A note from my journal at this time read, "… the Natren® probiotics appear to be more gentle at doing the job than Primal Defense® was at the same stage." I did have Herxheimer reactions, but I did not have the episodes of fierce urgency, or the degree of forceful movements as I did while on Primal Defense®.

I continued on in my regimen, increasing my Megadophilus® and Bifido Factor® powders by half a teaspoon weekly. If I noticed that bloating or cramping occurrences were too strong and/or lasted for more than three days, it was a signal that my body needed a little more time to adjust to the last dose; in that case, I would cut back to that previous dose for the rest of the week. After a week, and if I was feeling good, I chose to move up by a quarter teaspoon instead of half a teaspoon. I needed to make these smaller increases only a couple of times in the early weeks, but obviously, it points up a big advantage to using the powders. I continued gradually increasing my dosage until I reached four and a half teaspoons of each per day, which took me exactly five months.

At this point, I had built up my probiotic concentration enough that I was ready to try the Healthy Trinity® 3-in-1 capsule. I discontinued taking the powders and just took one 3-in-1 capsule with unchilled spring water during breakfast. Not only was it more convenient to take with food, my transition to the capsule was smooth; I had no adverse reactions or regression. However, after a month of staying at this dosage, I was unable to obtain further improvements, so I chose to increase to two 3-in-1 capsules per day.

Since I'd be doubling a very large dosage, I decided to make this adjustment slowly. It took me two weeks to work up to two capsules per day, and I found that pace was comfortable for me. The first week, I added the second capsule every other day at my last snack of the day. The second week, I alternated two days with two capsules, and one day without. During this time, I had a few Herxheimer reactions each week, and some occasional bloating. By the time I got to the third week, my body could handle two capsules a day without much bloating or discomfort.

Noticeable improvements came during the first week at two 3-in-1 capsules per day. Here, my health took a major upswing; my energy and clarity increased, and my bathroom trips were down to just three or four per day. I still experienced a few Herxheimer reactions, but they were becoming less challenging and only added a few more bathroom trips on those days.

I was so encouraged by my progress that after a week at two capsules per day I decided to try three; gradually working up to it over two weeks. During this time, I had a few Herxheimer reactions and some bloating, like I did at two capsules. After the first week at three capsules per day (one capsule at breakfast, lunch, and dinner), I was elated to notice even more improvements. This three capsule amount marked a giant leap forward in my health again. Now, I was really beginning to feel almost "normal." My energy and clarity were the highest they'd ever been. Bathroom trips were down to just two or three per day. Herxheimer reactions dwindled again, and the ones I had were minor, usually just a little headache or a few looser stools.

I tried moving up to four capsules a day gradually as I had done before, but I started to get Herxheimer reactions (mostly increased bathroom trips, and headaches) almost daily. When the symptoms did not subside after three weeks, I decided that this dose might be too much for my body. I dropped back down to three 3-in-1 capsules per day and within two weeks, my body returned to the excellent results I had previously at the three capsule dosage. In this way, I had discovered that three 3-in-1 capsules was the right goal dosage for me. After three months at this dosage, I experienced another major health gain.

A sample from my journal at this time reads,

"I feel like I'm well again! Even though the stools aren't absolutely perfect yet, they are more than good enough; my body really feels normal. I feel strong. Now, I only need the bathroom for less than five minutes just once or twice a day with no pain, blood, urgency or diarrhea. That's a far cry from the marathon twenty-plus times I used to go; it's like night and day!"

I was satisfied; even if I never got any better I could live the rest of my life like this and be happy. How could I complain? I felt normal, like there was nothing I couldn't do. I had energy and enthusiasm like I used to. But the best part was, I was still improving! I intend to stay at three 3-in-1 capsules per day until my stools are perfect, and then I will wean down to a maintenance dose of one capsule per day.

Final Thoughts on the Trials

On the right probiotics, long flare-ups were replaced by short adjustment days (a.k.a. Herxheimer reactions) until they dwindled in severity and number. These days usually included increased bathroom trips and brief periods of my old symptoms. Sometimes I also experienced sour stomach, bloating, acid reflux, increased appetite, headache, and/or slight fever. But they were all just passing minor discomforts and symbolized to me that significant changes were taking place. By keeping that in mind, it helped me not to over analyze any Herxheimer reactions; I learned that a fast way to discouragement was to judge every trip I had to the bathroom. So, on those adjustment days that I would need the toilet more, instead of getting discouraged, I tried to see it as my body taking another step toward improving. But if I were having excessive discomfort, or daily Herxheimer reactions for a week, it would be a signal to me that I best cut back on my dosage temporarily. On my program, it was important to remember that changes in my body were taking place constantly. And though I was tempted to speed up the process and increase my probiotic dosage more quickly, it was always best to give my body the necessary time to make those adjustments so that I would be more comfortable. I learned to go slow, feel good, and not to rush it.

Each of my successful trials showed that progress was being made even when it didn't show up in the toilet; the key was to never lose sight of the big picture. On the weeks that I didn't see improvement showing in the toilet, I almost always felt a gain in overall wellness and/or energy and thus, happiness. Whether it was by the day, the week, or the month, progress of some type was definitely being made. It was clear to me that I was succeeding by staying the course, steady and deliberate. I always felt like even a small improvement was improvement nonetheless. Some weeks there were more improvements, some not as many. But when I reviewed my journal notes over a month's time, progress was apparent.

Not only was choosing the right probiotics essential for progress, the amount was also. In Trial #13 for example, I discovered that one 3-in-1 capsule per day was insufficient to continue my progress after a month. I needed to get to two capsules per day to see my progress continue. Stools improved greatly at that dosage, and it was a good reminder that progress can stall if the proper dosage is not achieved. I gained even greater results after I worked up to three capsules per day. After three months at that dosage, my bathroom trips had decreased to just once or twice a day, what my doctor considers in the normal range. I tried to get to four capsules per day, but my body was better at three; I had found my max. The point is, that the benefits of the probiotics could not be fully realized if I didn't find my max. Too much I could always come down from, but too little wouldn't do enough. My trials convinced me that not all probiotics are created equal, and that the specific strains and amounts of these probiotics may play a big factor in overcoming this disease of the intestines.

My trials also proved that my body did not heal on its own. It responded to the successful regimen of diet, probiotics and medication. If any part of the successful regimen was removed, my progress was halted. The SCD™ kept the "bad" carbohydrates at a minimum and cleared the way for the probiotics to do their job of re-establishing a healthy flora and chasing out the pathogens. Likewise, my medication (Pentasa®) was invaluable in keeping the inflammation down so that the probiotics could promote healing. I could not heal without all three.

As you read here, this long battle consumed me completely for eight years. My motivation of refusing to stay sick proved to be a mighty one. Many of my trials were long, and almost all of them had very frustrating times. But, by having to repeat this program again and again, I became very experienced at what healing should feel like. I also proved that if it worked once, it would work again. The end result of finding my winning program was nothing short of amazing, and worth the entire struggle. I have what I set out to get from this endeavor: my freedom. I trust the recording of this long battle proved to you that some things are worth fighting for. Shouldn't your health be at the top of that list? The following chapters detail the complete program I developed for my success. I hope that this documentation will make someone's journey far more abbreviated.

PART 3: The Gut Help™ Program

"I get much comfort and relief just knowing that I have my program. Instead of sitting around waiting, I am finally on a path that at least points OUT of this endless frustration and chronic pain. That's what gives me real hope everyday."

– Journal entry 7.20.2005

The Six Core Components

As discovered through my trials, my winning program is comprised of:

1) Motivation
2) Medication (Pentasa®)
3) The Specific Carbohydrate Diet™
4) Natren® Probiotic supplements
5) Exercise routine
6) Journals

See Trial #13 for my exact dosages of medication and supplements. The following sections detail my exact procedures and rules that I followed while on my program. They were all "battle-tested" over my eight years of trials, and subsequently, essential to my success.

1) Motivation

No one is happy that they have IBD or IBS. But that frustration was all I needed to motivate me in the right direction: the search for a way out. I was angry. I hated living in the prison of this relentless illness. I was truly sick of being sick. After twelve years, I finally accepted how much I was losing; how this illness robbed me of my freedom and happiness. I had waited long enough for a magic pill; this illness was not getting better on it's own, and I was the one who was losing out everyday. While I may have accepted my sickness, I wasn't going to accept that nothing more could be done about it without surgery.

Instead of surrendering to my plight, I stopped playing the victim and let my frustration fuel my desire to help myself. It was time I played a more active role in my health. **I realized that I would never have the life I wanted if I kept allowing myself to suffer the way I was.** That was the huge first step I needed, and essentially the first building block of my program.

A shift had been made. Now I wanted to change more than anything else. I was not going to stand in the way of my progress; I was not going to let myself down. It was just a matter of doing whatever was necessary to try and make my dream a reality. And that's how I started taking ownership of my health. My healing experience has taught me that in some ways, changing careers is harder than changing my life with this illness. There is much logic in my healing program - there aren't many things in life that are so straightforward.

As you read in my trials, finding the diet was just the beginning. To make my program yield the big improvements I was looking for, I had to add and subtract foods, medications, and supplements until I got it right. That took time. But the motivation I developed was so powerful that it kept me focused and determined, even through the years of setbacks and disappointments I endured. I owe my eventual success almost completely to it; it kept me committed the entire way.

2) Medication

Trial #10 proved that my medication, Pentasa®, was necessary to keep my inflammation down during healing. My doctor told me that Pentasa® was best taken with food, so I made it easy to remember by taking my 1000mg dosage three times a day at mealtimes, or just after.

3) The Specific Carbohydrate Diet™

The diet I followed was from the book by Elaine Gottschall, *Breaking the Vicious Cycle*. It details the foods permitted on the Specific Carbohydrate Diet™ as well as the science behind it. Basically, I stayed away from all milk, wheat, rice, soy, disaccharide sugars, difficult to digest starches, and any products made with these ingredients. The book contains important details that are essential to understand. It would not be wise to begin this diet without reading her book, and first discussing it with your gastroenterologist and a nutritionist.

If I ever had any suspicions about a particular food item that was not mentioned in her book, I'd try to research it by clicking on the "Legal list" link at: www.breakingtheviciouscycle.info Here you'll find an up to date alphabetical list of the foods allowed and not allowed on the diet.

Starting the Diet

Getting used to the SCD™ is a lot like driving a car with manual transmission – once you get it, you never forget it. At first you have to think about shifting, and then after a while, it becomes second nature. Everything I ate was approved on the diet, and I stuck to the diet fanatically. If I needed to eat and had no safe food available, I would go to the grocery store and get what I needed. I would never use the lack of safe food as an excuse to cheat. Never. I knew the only person I'd be cheating would be me. I was sick of being sick and I wanted to get well as fast as I could. So cheating was out!

Almost always I ate three moderate size meals a day with three good size snacks. I'd have one snack before lunch, one before dinner, and almost always, one before 9pm. I was usually getting hungry around 8:30 PM and I didn't want to be starving when I went to bed a few hours later. The last snack was usually very small. The following are my diet survival rules that came from much experience.

Steve's Top Ten Diet Survival Rules:

1) I never eat after 9 PM, unless it's a dire emergency. This took a little practice, but it was the smart thing to do. It gave my intestines a much-needed evening break to

rest and promote healing.

2) Limit soda intake. No more than two diet sodas a week. No sugar soda. Otherwise, I made my own "juice cocktails" freely. I preferred these instead of diet soda. I used 100% natural OJ or Welch's 100% purple grape juice (from bottle only, not the can) and mixed it with seltzer water or club soda (about 20% juice, 80% club soda). Juice cocktails are delicious and much more nutritious than diet soda. However, there were times when a diet soda was the perfect complement to a meal, and so I'd save it for those occasions.

3) Limit alcohol intake. Only two glasses of dry red or white wine per week. No beer. Occasionally, I'd substitute a scotch, gin, rye or bourbon only. I never drank heavily, but like most folks, I did enjoy relaxing with a few drinks on the right occasion. So on the program, I now had to plan how many and where (if at all) I was going to have my two drinks. It was challenging at first, but not impossible. I just had to re-think how I drank socially, putting the emphasis on the time I was having, rather than the "buzz" from a few more drinks. This was an important rule to follow, for if I didn't, I'd get increased symptoms (especially diarrhea, cramps, soreness, and even some bleeding) the next day or two. It was definitely not worth the pain and discomfort to disregard this rule.

4) No sugar or any of its derivatives like high fructose corn syrup, or evaporated cane juice. I stayed away from all gum (sugarless or otherwise) and over-the-counter medications unless prescribed by my doctor. Most of these contained sugar, cornstarch, or forms of sugar such as aspartame, sorbitol, manitol or xylitol, all of which are not allowed on the diet. The only sweet I allow in my body is 100% pure honey (a simple sugar, and therefore SCD™ safe) or the natural sugar in fresh fruits. (To be diet safe, I also had a compounding pharmacist make me a prescription of filler and binder free acetaminophen capsules for any occasional headaches I'd get.)

5) The only flour I eat is almond flour. I never eat any other flours, batters or coatings, wheat, corn, oat or otherwise. Never.

6) Never eat soy products or soy sauce. That goes for tofu and soybeans too. Soy sauce is fermented wheat, and that's just about the single worst thing I can possibly eat for my condition.

7) Never eat rice or potatoes of any variety. Obviously, I never eat derivatives of these like cornstarch, potato starch, or modified food starch of any kind.

8) Always take a snack when I'm away from home. I prefer something portable and quick such as fresh fruit, homemade nut-mix, or an almond flour cookie so I won't be caught without a safe choice between meals. In the early stages of the diet when cramps and soreness were more active, I had to be much more cautious about not eating too many nuts during the course of a day.

9) Never eat anything at a restaurant or a party when I don't know the exact ingredients or the preparation method. Eating out was never an excuse for me to lose ground on my program. If it isn't on the diet, I don't eat it. I never feel bad asking about a food because so many people have food allergies and strict diets these days.

10) Use the site. If I ever had any suspicions about a particular food item, I looked it up in either the book, *Breaking the Vicious Cycle*, or at the official book website. Click on the "Legal list" link at: www.breakingtheviciouscycle.info

Staying with the Diet

Preparing my SCD™ safe food was challenging at first, but I knew it was worth it; I was now helping myself instead of hurting. Unlike my previous unhealthy take-out lifestyle, it was time-consuming to have to cook, but my health was definitely worth it. Soon I began to really enjoy it; I found it relaxing and discovered I wasn't alone. Savvy people everywhere are rediscovering the joy of cooking and eating together as an alternative to the more expensive, and often less nutritious, take-out lifestyle that is marketed to us all. To my surprise, cooking improved the quality of my life in more ways than one.

Main dishes were easier to prepare. I preferred chicken, pork or fish, fresh from the store, and cooked in olive oil and herbs without any soy, wheat, rice or sugar. When desired, I used blanched almond flour as a substitute for a healthier and diet safe bread crumb-like coating.

I enjoyed shopping at Whole Foods (a health conscious grocery store chain) during the week. Since I didn't have a lot of time but I needed fresh ingredients, I usually would make two quick grocery store trips per week: one for meats, fish and poultry for entrées, and the other for fresh fruits and veggies. It was fun to experiment with new recipes and entrée/vegetable combinations. I'd usually spend part of Sundays just baking the goods I'd need for the next week or two. That was a great weekday time saver tip, courtesy of my favorite cook… my mom!

Cravings were the first hurdle I had to overcome when I started the diet. And the first thing I needed was a sweet and satisfying cookie, something that could take the place of my mad cravings for chocolate chip cookies. It was crucial to my success to get this recipe going right away. So mom and I made an almond flour cookie with flakes of unsweetened coconut, raisins, walnuts, and honey. It was delicious! In fact, it was so satisfying for a sweet fix that I made and ate that cookie exclusively for one whole year! (Yes, it was that good.) I loved that cookie at all hours of the day. It was really satisfying for breakfast in the beginning of the diet if I had an extra sweet tooth that morning (with some fruit and cheese of course). After one year, I tried other great variations like pecan cookies, coconut cookies and more. Eventually, my desire for these cookies at breakfast tapered off once I began making my amazing cheddar cheese pancakes (see Part 8, Favorite Recipes). Finally I didn't feel left out anymore; I could now have "pancakes" like all the people I was envious of in the diner.

Other giant breakthroughs that made the diet easier to stay on were making my own chips and focaccia bread (see Part 8, Favorite Recipes). The chips are made from thinly sliced butternut squash, and deep-fried. Once I bought a good food processor, the right thin blade, and a big deep fryer, I was in heaven. When in season, fried butternut squash chips taste better than any potato chips; they have more flavor, nutrition, and obviously, are not as harmful to my gut. I made sure to fry them in only canola oil so they were even healthier than any chip on the market.

My almond flour focaccia bread was my ultimate versatile diet safe bread. I'd love it just toasted and dunked in olive oil, just like all the delicious Italian breads you'd get at a restaurant. This bread was the key to making my day taste great; now I had absolutely no reason to feel deprived! I could have it at breakfast with eggs, make an egg sandwich, or use it for French toast. At lunch it made the best sandwiches that never fell apart, or at dinner I could toast it and use it for bruschetta. It even made a terrific pizza crust; the list goes on and on. I'm now experimenting with making sun-dried tomato focaccia bread.

After two months on the diet, I no longer felt the severe addict-like cravings for refined sugar or bread that I once had. My discipline had paid off. I had successfully detoxed my taste buds and the mental habits of always thinking and reaching for sugar or bread snacks. This was a huge milestone. I felt so empowered, like I was Superman. And in a way, I guess I was. I had done something I never thought I could do, and in turn it gave me confidence like I never had.

At this point, I was able to eat less of my cookies per day and greatly appreciate the natural sweet satisfying taste of fruits. All the ones I never used to eat like plums, nectarines, peaches and more. Soon, fruit became my favorite dessert. There's nothing like cherries that are in season for real taste-bud satisfaction. I couldn't believe it; I was actually enjoying – even craving – fruit for the very first time in my life! It was so much more satisfying than refined sugar and all the more delicious because it was so good for me. Now I was giving my body what it really needed, essential vitamins, nutrients and fiber that only come from fruit. I began to understand the prison that refined sugar had me trapped in. And worst of all, refined sugar's hyper-sweetness dissuaded me from eating the good foods my body needed, like fruit. Not anymore!

Soon, I learned to always have quick-foods on hand, to use as a safe go-to when I was too tired, or not in the mood to cook a fresh meal for dinner. My favorites were canned tuna (packed in only olive oil and salt, no added starches) and frozen almond flour pizza. I'd make a batch of almond flour pizza once a month (in two big rectangle baking trays) and then freeze it. This way, whenever the pizza craving hit me, I could just get it from the freezer and enjoy it with the same convenience as regular frozen pizza. Then I could rest and take the evening off, feel like everyone else, and get to the grocery more leisurely the next day. Safe go-to foods put a lot of normalcy back in my life.

Variety is the key to sticking with any diet. But because the consequences were greater if I slipped off the diet, variety played even more of an important role in keeping me satisfied. I learned that the trick to staying happy on the diet for me was that I varied my meals and leftovers before I got bored. I got used to thinking a week ahead. This way, it was far less likely that I'd get bummed-out and miss my old favorite foods if I always kept something new to look forward to. I knew if I was enjoying coconut cookies this week, I might want to try pecan cookies the next. Or if I had leftovers of chicken for two days, I should get creative with the leftover prep, like use tomato sauce (all natural, no sugar added) or make a stir-fry.

To keep the variety going, I'd get inspired watching cooking shows on the Food Network and then I'd alter the recipes for my diet. Only one or two different recipes or tricks for leftovers were needed. It was a great way to keep up my positive attitude and enthusiasm, while also fun and good for my health. I wrote down and saved my favorite new recipes to use when I needed a change in the future. It was amazing how my library of interesting dishes multiplied and kept me from getting the blahs; that's something I couldn't say even before I was on the diet.

4) Natren® Probiotic Supplements

See Trial #13 for exact dosages. Also, please make sure to read my final thoughts on the trials; there is very valuable insight about my probiotic experience contained therein.

After five months, when I switched from the Natren® powders to the 3-in-1 capsules, I had to change my schedule slightly. The 3-in-1 capsule should be taken with food, so I usually took it in the middle of my meal, and then I'd wait to take my Pentasa® at the end of the meal. This schedule worked very well for me.

At two capsules per day, I was taking one in the morning, and one at night. When I got up to three capsules per day, I took one with each meal - breakfast, lunch, and dinner. Spreading the capsules throughout the day gave me the best results. I did also take an SCD™ one-a-day multivitamin manufactured by Freeda Vitamins, usually after breakfast. See more of my routines in their separate section later in this chapter.

5) Exercise

Journal entry from ten months into Trial #13:

After being away from the gym over the weekend I was feeling a bit lethargic, but I knew I was rested and able to workout. I made the effort to get to the gym and now that I'm back, I'm so glad that I went. I feel 100% better than I did an hour ago! What a difference in my energy and spirit after a good twenty-minute jog, I'm much more alive and awake. This is what exercising gives me; it's where I get my positivity and fuels my spirit's strength.

As you could probably guess, exercise was a favorite part of my program. There was a noticeable improvement in my overall well-being once I started exercising even a little. And as I healed, I naturally wanted to exercise more. I discovered that exercise is a rare addiction that is actually good for you. Everyone knows regular exercise helps us stay fit, lower our cholesterol and strengthen our bodies, but that's just the beginning. Once after an ear infection, I learned of the power of exercise when my doctor prescribed light walking to help me boost my immune system. It helped speed my recovery, my concentration and focus. After a cautious start, I knew it belonged in my program; it does wonders for my positive attitude, which kept me even more committed to my program for success. As an added bonus, it got me outside which was where I wanted to be. Without a doubt, exercise helped me greatly, but I had to start slowly.

I had to remember that heavy physical activity was going to make me exhausted and take away from my body's most important efforts to heal my gut. My golden rule for exercise was that I would only do it if I felt rested and strong enough. I never exercised on flare-up or Herxheimer reaction days where I might notice blood, or if I was exhausted. It was much better to listen to my body and take that day off to rest because that's what I needed more. On the days I felt well enough, I did what ever I could do comfortably, never pushing.

Nothing said "I'm getting better" more to me than being outside. Once I felt better, I also tried biking and rollerblading to change things up, but again, never working out hard or for longer than twenty minutes of cardio. I wanted to wait until my gut completely healed before I pushed it harder. It just made sense.

My Exercise Methods

During the first three months of the program, I did not exercise. This allowed me to focus on healing without adding physical stress. It also was smart to give myself time to get used to the new diet and the weekly probiotic increases. Once I got an understanding for how my body reacted to those increases (i.e., seeing the pattern in my bathroom trips) I was ready to get some exercise outside. The primary reason for my exercising wasn't to put heavy strain on my body and challenge myself like a competition weightlifter or marathon runner – hardly! It was just for the simple joy of feeling good from a little workout. Nothing big. It was more for my mind than it was for my body – that was the key. I found all other aspects of my life (concentration, energy, and the most important, positive attitude) benefited from just a short simple workout.

My first exercise workout was just a simple walk around my street. I chose a time that was well after my daily bathroom trips so it wouldn't be likely that I'd need to go again. That gave me confidence. I walked no more than ten minutes at a very relaxed pace. I was in no rush and didn't put any pressure on myself to set any records. I was doing this just for the joy of being outside; it was celebrating the gift of freedom, something I couldn't do before without fear. For that reason alone, this first short walk/test was a breakthrough success for my spirit. It was so wonderful to focus on the sound of the gravel beneath my feet and the smell of the air, instead of worrying if I'd need to run home for the bathroom. I was amazed at how grateful I felt to be free for those ten minutes.

Now I was hooked.

I came home, and rested that afternoon, and "checked-in" with myself to see how the walk affected me. I felt good, strong and positive, not winded or tired. Though I was tempted, I chose not to push it and waited to the next day to see if I felt up to doing it again. I did. And that's how I started putting exercise in my program. At that time, the only criteria I had for going out to walk was: did I have a break in bathroom trips? And was I too tired? Some weeks I walked two days in a row then one day off. Others, I walked one day, then rested one or two. I just did it according to how I felt.

As the month went on and my healing and energy increased, I naturally wanted to walk longer; I was ready for fifteen minutes a day. After another month, twenty minutes a day. That was my limit. I tried not to walk more than twenty minutes without a rest. As my confidence increased, I was able to drive to different parks much farther from my home, and a bathroom! I'd meet up with friends, or take my dog on a little nature walk. All of these things I did to celebrate my ever increasing freedom that my program was affording me. This was what I had been waiting for.

I also enjoyed adding a low intensity Yoga program (no more than twenty minutes) at home on rainy days, or when I wanted a change from walking. Yoga made me feel incredible from the very first time I tried it. Even after just fifteen minutes of basic positions and simple relaxation exercises, I could feel improvement in my posture and alertness for the rest of the day. Yoga also allowed me to stimulate different muscle groups that walking didn't, and that offered a beneficial type of cross training to my weekly routine. Had I found Yoga earlier, I might have tried it before walking outside because it affords an extra peace of mind by being in the comfort of home, that is, close to a bathroom if I needed it.

After six months and a successful transition to the Healthy Trinity® 3-in-1 oil matrix pill, I was in a comfortable period (regular, predictable bathroom trips) and ready to try some light weightlifting for strength building. I found that like walking, I didn't need to push it so hard to gain benefits of mind and body. I joined a gym (another freedom I hadn't enjoyed before) and found a trainer. I explained my health condition to him, and he began to educate me on proper lifting technique. After a month of training a few times a week, I had created a good program that I still follow. It contained just a few simple exercises for my major muscle groups that I could easily complete in about twenty minutes.

This small addition of lightweight resistance training did many positive things for my life. It built strength of my muscles but most important, it built strength of my mind – a crucial ally that I needed in my fight against this illness. These new positive feelings about my life and my healing seemed to coincide in perfect unison with the results of my diet and probiotic regimen. They all worked together for an incredible positive high that made me psyched to continue. That's how I knew I had a wonderful program; simultaneously it was healing my mind, body and spirit. I didn't hate my body anymore; I began to respect it. I now looked forward to weightlifting instead of dreading it.

Timing my eating and exercising was important. I tried to time my workouts so that I was exercising about an hour to an hour and a half after I had eaten. The diet limits my carbohydrates, so I need to eat more often than people not on the diet. It wasn't a big deal to work around once I figured out my eating schedule and when I got hungry. Then it was just a matter of exercising after I had enough time to digest my last meal (usually an hour) and before the next time I'd get hungry. This technique would carry me through my short workout without fear of running out of energy and risking exhaustion. I want to be comfortable when I exercise, therefore, I never exercise less than an hour after I eat. The following is an example workout of mine from seven months into my program.

Weekly Exercise Example
7 months into The Gut Help™ Program

It's just plain common sense - never attempt this or any exercise program without first consulting your physician and a professional physical trainer. It was critical that I worked with a trainer to learn proper technique, and the right exercises for me.

This example was worked up to gradually and only attempted after seven months on The Gut Help™ Program, after I had already achieved a dosage of two Natren® Healthy Trinity® 3-in-1 capsules per day.

I started with very low weights for all exercises, gradually increasing every two or three weeks if I felt strong and ready. I always practiced proper technique to avoid injury, and I never strained on any of the reps. If I felt tired, I decreased the weight or stopped the activity for the day. I wanted to only stimulate the muscle - never put a heavy load on it. My goal was to increase my energy and stimulate my immune system, not get exhausted!

Once I reached a comfortable level of medium weights, I did not go higher. Then, every two or three weeks I'd just change the exercises to keep my muscles stimulated and growing. This was only after I really got a good understanding of the variety of exercises and how they worked for each muscle group from my trainer. I looked forward to making the changes, mixing and matching different exercises to make a fun workout. I still did not do more than two exercises per muscle group. After exercising, if I felt I needed another day of rest, I just took the day off and moved the whole schedule up a day.

Monday: **Chest and Triceps day**
2 Chest exercises, 3 sets of each
2 Triceps exercises, 3 sets of each

Tuesday: **Cardio**
I would choose only one of the following: walk 20 minutes, or 20 minutes of Yoga, or 20 minutes of elliptical machine or light jog if feeling really good.

Wednesday: **Back and Biceps day**
2 Back exercises, 3 sets of each
2 Bicep exercises, 3 sets of each

Thursday: **Cardio**
Here I'd choose another cardio activity from Tuesday's list, only one, for 20 minutes.

Friday: **Shoulders and Legs day**
2 Shoulders exercises, 3 sets of each
2 Legs exercises, 3 sets of each

Saturday: **Off**
Sunday: **Off**

As you can see, I never did cardio (i.e., walk or run) on the same day I would lift. After much experimentation I discovered that it was just too much strain to put on myself while on the road to healing. It was also important to take the weekend off and get my rest. That kept my energy from running too low, and also got me psyched to work out on Monday. Occasionally, if family was together or my dog needed to get out more, I'd do a short additional walk on the weekend. But for the most part, I liked to do other activities with friends, or catch up on playing guitar. This became a little more challenging when I started to feel better and wanted to do more. But I just remembered to preserve my energy and always do a little less than I thought I could; that worked well for me.

I kept my enthusiasm and motivation high by having an easy number of exercises I knew I could get through. I think that was a great idea and the real reason I got psyched for lifting; it was just the right amount of exercise with an end in sight. It wasn't a huge time commitment either; I could do it in a half hour or less usually. And I always felt great after. That's when I knew I had it right.

I look forward to my weightlifting every week, even now. I know it plays a large roll in keeping my energy, strength, enthusiasm, and positivity very high. I feel as if my body needs it; and I have learned, it really does. I just needed to create the right exercise program for my condition.

6) Journals

I have kept two journals since I started my trials in 1998. One journal is just to record my daily food consumption and bathroom trips, and the other is a personal journal to record my thoughts and feelings. Each of these played an integral role in my program, and in more ways than one, greatly helped me succeed.

My wife easily created these journals on her computer with a program called FileMaker Pro (see examples at the end of this section). Since these journals were on a computer, all of my entries could be done neatly and quickly. If you wanted to start journaling right away on paper, you could follow the same format as my examples. A plain white sheet of paper, a notebook, or a loose-leaf notebook, would all work. An obvious advantage to having my journals computerized was that it allowed me to quickly search for keywords at any time. This made tracking food allergies, and the effectiveness of probiotics, much easier. I could see progress over time, a very important advantage that turned into a necessity for discovering my program.

The layout for the journals was simple. Each day was kept to a single page, with separate sections created specifically for each journal. For example, in the food journal, there were sections to write in what I had for breakfast, lunch, and dinner with separate sections in between each to log snacks. There was also a large notes section where I would log how many times I went to the bathroom that day and what the results were.

Keeping journals had other advantages too. By writing everything I ate for the first six months of my program, I was able to see how I was adapting to the diet. It allowed me to recognize eating patterns, and quickly get a handle on bad eating habits (e.g., noshing on too many nuts during the day, or noticing which food group I wasn't eating enough from). These were important observations that I was only able to spot quickly and correct because I was diligent in keeping and reviewing my journal.

Since I wrote in the food journal everyday, I didn't want it to become a long and tedious task to dread. That's why I developed my own shorthand system. This allowed me to quickly recap what happened during my daily bathroom trips with symbols instead of long phrases. For example, if I had diarrhea I typed the letter "D." If my stool was formed I typed "S" for solid, if it was loose, I'd type "L." I also had other symptoms I wanted abbreviations for, like "C" for cramps, "SP" for spasms, "B" for blood, "U" for urgency, and "P" for pain. I liked to use the + or − symbols next to the letters to indicate "more" or "less" if it was applicable. For example, lots of cramps would be C+, while very slight cramps would be C-.

Every time I needed the toilet, I made sure to also enter the time of day. This allowed me to quickly spot changes in daily patterns when I'd need the toilet most often (invaluable information for planning my outside activities accordingly). Sometimes, I also used short phrases if I wanted to remark about something new or unusual that a symbol couldn't quite say. For example, "felt stronger today," or "had more energy" would be just enough telling detail for future reference.

My symbols and notations were all very helpful to me as they simplified progress analysis. For example, if I wanted to know if my cramps had decreased over a month's time, I would search back to the first week of the month and count how many times I wrote the letter C (for cramps) per day. Then, I'd take an average of that number to arrive at the average number of cramps per day in the first week of the month. I'd do the same for the last week of the month and then compare the two numbers. I often did this for many of my symptoms to track their progress. This actually was fun and exciting; especially when there was dramatic improvement.

After six months of food journaling, when I felt like I really understood the diet and making the right food choices, I decided to stop writing down everything I ate and let myself simply enjoy my new life. This was a great idea for me, as it brought less focus on the diet and my differences from others, and highlighted the fact that I was still a person, like everyone else. *I did not stop writing down all my bathroom trips, however. And I never stopped eating the SCD™ way.*

The personal journal was my place to write whatever I wanted. It only needed two sections, one for a date, and the other a big space to write my thoughts. If I was angry or grumpy, then I wrote it. If I was happy and optimistic, then I wrote that too. This journal was only about what I was feeling, and it was great therapy just for that. It seemed more like a traditional journal. I wrote what was important to me at the time; it could be comments about family trips, daily life, my gut, or not. It was my place to be validated. And over time, it helped me examine my fears and doubts, eventually, refocusing them into strength and courage.

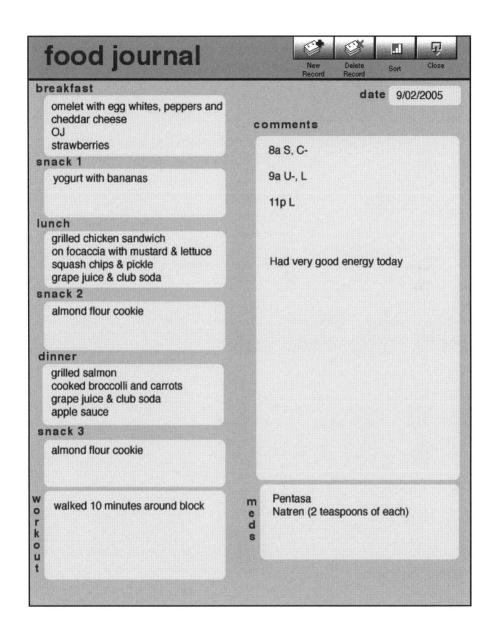

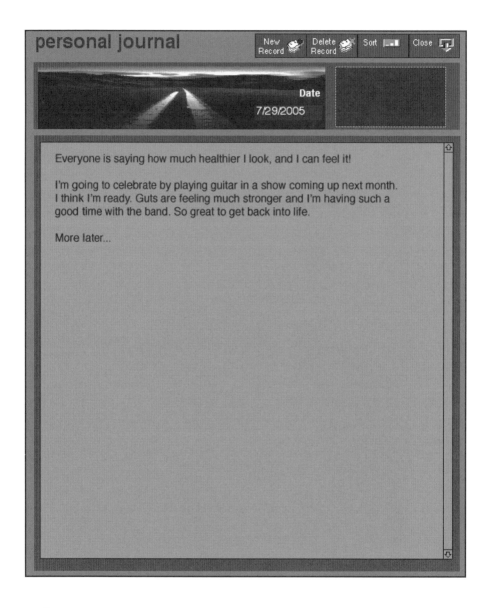

personal journal   New Record   Delete Record   Sort   Close

Date
7/29/2005

Everyone is saying how much healthier I look, and I can feel it!

I'm going to celebrate by playing guitar in a show coming up next month. I think I'm ready. Guts are feeling much stronger and I'm having such a good time with the band. So great to get back into life.

More later...

The Gut Help™ Program Routines

My Gut Help™ Program required consistency to be effective. I quickly discovered the many benefits from keeping a routine. Most notably, it provided me comfort and confidence, especially when I was facing the challenge of healing my gut. A routine was definitely needed because there were many elements I had to juggle by day and by week. After some trial and error, I found a way to balance my cooking and eating routines to fit nicely with my medication and supplement routines. What follows are the methods I used.

Cooking Routine

At first I just cooked whenever I needed to, but it didn't take long before this "method" (or lack thereof) became impractical. A better solution for me was to make a cooking schedule. Slowly, I was building a library of favorite recipes that I could pick from. Then, I'd choose one day a week (usually Sunday) and prepare the baked items or any entrées I needed for the coming week. For example, not only would I bake bread and cookies, I'd make several baked chicken breasts so I could have one with veggies for dinner one night; another in a salad the next day, another in a sandwich with my bread, and still another with homemade tomato sauce later in the week. I could do the same with beef or lamb, and have even more options for the week. I also would make a batch of pizza with my focaccia bread (see Part 8, Favorite Recipes) and freeze it, so I could have it on hand if I got too tired to cook during the coming week. Whenever I needed a change, usually two or three times a week, I could pick up some fresh fish (always a tasty, healthy addition to my diet), add some fresh or microwaved frozen veggies (diet safe only), and this meal was ready fast.

Preparing foods ahead of time was the key to my convenience and variety during the workweek. I always felt more normal when I could just reach into the fridge and make a safe, fast meal; that was priceless to me. Instantly, I could nourish my body, stay on track with my healing progress, and still feel like "everyone else" at the same time. It also gave me the ability to enjoy more quality free time instead of always being in the kitchen. Now that's cookin'!

Supplement, Medicine and Eating Routines

My probiotic supplement and medicine routine helped me easily fall into a comfortable eating routine. When I was taking the probiotic powders, it all got started with my morning dose, twenty minutes before breakfast with unchilled spring water. The rest of the day then consisted of three major meals (breakfast, lunch and dinner) with three interspersed snacks. I took my prescribed dosage of medication (1000mg Pentasa®) with each major meal. My second and last dose of probiotic powder for the day came twenty minutes before dinner with unchilled spring water. After I had made the transition to the Natren® 3-in-1 Healthy Trinity® capsule, I began taking them with food as recommended. I would take my 3-in-1 capsule with unchilled spring water at the beginning of the meal, and take the Pentasa at the end.

It served me well to have a balanced meal for each of my major meals. I preferred slightly favoring protein and vegetables, but I'd make sure to also get a serving of dairy (some kind of safe cheese or yogurt), a serving of almond flour bread or cookie, and a fruit portion if needed. Because I followed the rule of no food after 9 PM, I was very hungry when I awoke. *I never skipped a meal because each one provided me with the necessary energy to get to the next.* If I skipped a meal, I would become weak and tired, unable to function to my best ability. So I learned to put down my work when it was time to eat, and eat. Food is energy! The effort I was making to heal would've been greatly hindered if I did not stop to get my body the fuel it needed.

I would eat a snack because usually I was hungry about an hour to an hour and a half after each major meal. This would give me enough time to have an empty stomach for my evening dose of probiotic powder before dinner. The twenty minutes I'd wait after taking my probiotics was also a perfect time to make the meal. During dinner, I'd take my last dose of Pentasa® for the day. After the meal, I'd wait an hour or two and then have my last snack if I were still hungry.

I had no food after 9 PM, especially in the first six months. This gave my intestines a longer chance to rest and heal before the next day. The only time I'd eat after 9 PM was if it was a hunger "emergency" (headache or weakness induced), or if I had been traveling and was used to a different time zone, which I slowly adjusted back in a few days.

I found there was a nice rhythm to the day when I followed my supplement and eating routine closely. They worked well together and gave me a sense strength and progress. *One of the most important reasons that I established a routine was so that bowel function can begin to get regulated, and afford me more freedom ASAP!* Once the routine was established, I could almost predict when I'd have to go to the bathroom (no small wonder considering I could never do that before I started my program). That precious freedom granted meant I could leave the house with more confidence and return to a job, or fun activities away from home with less likelihood of an emergency. The day I realized I wasn't looking for the bathroom anymore was the day I knew I was on my way, a very happy day indeed. (See Part 7 for example meals and snacks.)

The Gut Help™ Lifestyle

Going Out to Eat

For the first month on my program I chose to stay home and make all my meals to get adjusted to the diet. I think that was a good call. Soon, I wanted a break from the cooking and felt like going out to eat. I was committed to the diet so I would not use going out as an excuse to cheat and order things like French fries; I could see the good my program was doing for me, and I did not want to stop it. I figured I could find something on most menus that was on the diet, but I had to stay alert.

When I got to a restaurant and opened the menu there were traps abound! Most main entrees had sauces and reductions that needed to be avoided. Yes, they all sounded good, but those sauces and reductions were most likely made with flour, starch, milk, sugar and/or soy – all mortal enemies of the diet, and thus, my mortal enemies. I would usually just choose another entrée or have them hold the sauce or reduction. If dishes were prepared with rice or potatoes, they were easily altered by asking for a substitution of cooked veggies, or a side salad with oil and red wine vinegar (never balsamic), or just lemon.

The first time out I thought I'd try something simple like steak. But later I found that even upset me because it must have been marinated in some kind of Worcestershire, or soy sauce. That was disheartening, and a set back that could have been avoided. It was a lesson I learned for the next time: always ask about the preparation! I shouldn't have felt ashamed or embarrassed about my condition or diet; *I was paying for the meal, and I should get it the way I want it.* Besides, almost everyone today is following special diets because of food allergies, or for other health reasons. Special orders are commonplace now; there is no reason to feel embarrassed.

I learned it pays to read the menu first, find something that's closest to the diet, then ask the waiter to make sure they will prepare it accordingly (i.e., no flour or breading, broiling a plain steak instead of marinating with sauce, cooking veggies in butter or olive oil instead of margarine, etc.). From the appetizer to a dessert course of fruit only, I found it pays not to guess, but to ask about all of it. I go out to eat for a happy change of scenery, not to lose ground on my road to recovery. And you really don't have to make a big deal of it and draw attention to yourself. I'd just usually say something like, "Hi, I'm on a special diet and I was wondering if you use any milk, flour, soy, or sugar in the preparation of this chicken dish." Or I'd say, "I have food allergies and I was wondering if you use any milk, flour, soy, or sugar in the preparation of this chicken dish." I preferred the latter. By saying I had a food allergy the waiter would always perk up and get serious, taking a keen interest in making my order exactly how I asked (most likely fearing that I would die if he brought me anything I told him not to). I usually didn't offer any other details and that was all it took for the waiter to give my request serious attention. The point is that it's more than just suggesting that you would prefer not to have an ingredient, it's stating clearly that you can not have an ingredient or something bad will happen, which was true for my gut. They don't have to know what, and they never ask. And that's what the food allergy description did for me.

It didn't take long to adjust to eating out on my program. Within a couple months I got the hang of it, and I was easily finding restaurants that were better suited for my diet. One of my favorites was a Greek restaurant that would make fresh grilled chicken kabobs. One day I asked a waiter about the preparation of the dishes that interested me, and I just remembered which ones he said were safe for future visits. Then, when ordering one of those dishes the next time, I could just say, "Hold the rice," and I knew that I was safe; that was nice and easy. The relaxation and convenience was a real lifesaver on those days that I was too tired to cook.

Restaurants that posed the biggest threat to my diet were fast food chains, as well as Chinese and Indian food restaurants. At fast food chain restaurants, there was too much risk of bad starches and sugars being in absolutely everything, from the burgers to the salads. That "chicken" they put on fast food salads is the processed kind. The kind that's available in the prepared foods section of the grocery store and loaded with modified food starch and other diet no-nos. I avoided these restaurants at all costs, only considering eating the meat in a hamburger, or the lettuce from a salad (with no dressing) if it was an absolute emergency and I had no other restaurant choice, which wasn't often.

I seldom ate at Chinese food restaurants. Their fried food is loaded with flour, salt, soy, and food starch. Even the less noxious stir-fried dishes are loaded with salt and soy sauce. And yes, even the steamed chicken in most dishes has almost always been marinated in chicken broth that has modified food starch. Indian restaurants I avoided for their use of yogurt (not prepared according to the diet) in almost all dishes. I'm always suspecting sauces when I eat out. My safe rule of thumb is: if I didn't make the sauce, then I can't trust what's in it - no matter what some person behind the counter says. They may be forgetting something, even when I ask them directly; they don't really understand that even the slightest infraction makes it harder to heal. So that's why I avoided these kinds of restaurants, it was just too difficult to get a meal that wouldn't have some kind of infraction.

Developing a keen eye to spot dishes that looked like trouble and avoid them was a skill I built up fast. The caveat to eating out is that you have to trust what the waiter tells you about a dish. Experience taught me that can be a costly mistake. I would rather eat something boring and safe and not get sick, than take a chance and pay the price of a set back. I always told myself: no food tastes as good as freedom feels! I had to put my health first.

Soon, I discovered some safe favorites that I could quickly order when I didn't want to think too much while I was out. Namely, shrimp cocktail (just with lemon, no red sauce), plain grilled steak, plain grilled hamburger (no bun) with only real cheddar cheese and yellow mustard, plain grilled or broiled chicken and fish (prepared with just butter, lemon, and fresh herbs), and cooked or steamed veggies in olive oil or butter only. And for salad, I'd have it with just olive oil and lemon, or red wine vinegar, no balsamic vinegar. Salads at quality restaurants are one of the easiest things to get right on the diet, but they should be avoided when having a flare-up, or a Hercheimer reaction day. For those times, I made other choices temporarily, like fish or meat with cooked veggies, or I just made sure not to eat too much salad.

Early on, I noticed that going out to eat could cause feelings of temptation and/or guilt. This is just natural because I had to say a difficult goodbye to some of my favorite foods. Changing my habits wouldn't happen overnight, but I can say it's been well worth it. When I first tried the diet, I did feel frustration when I was at a mall food court and saw people eating my old favorite, pizza! These natural feelings passed as I learned to make my own satisfying pizza and saw the health gains from my program. Best of all, I never had any temptations after the first two months on my program. That's a fact straight from an ex-pizza eating, chocolate chip cookie lovin', and cola-gulping madman.

Helping Myself

I achieved great success during my program by learning to pay closer attention to my body and its needs. In this way, I was really helping myself. This is much different from how I used to think; I was now taking ownership of my health. I became my own protector, and nobody knew me better than me.

If I were getting "the blahs" from my food choices, I'd look to cook books or food shows on TV to give me new ideas for basic recipes that I could alter. If I were feeling a little down from work, but I knew I still had some energy, I'd make time to get outside and exercise. I used simple common sense solutions like these to keep myself happy on my road to recovery. That was the big picture I didn't want to lose sight of.

I tried never to sit with my problems for too long, and I got very quick at tuning into my needs. This was a healthy habit, and a replacement for turning to chocolate or junk food to make myself feel better like I used to. I was teaching myself to be strong and to problem solve, to move from being a victim to being a victor. Finding time for good friends and a supportive therapist who validated my efforts was also a smart way in which I helped myself.

On the Job with The Gut Help™ Program

By the third month on my program, I began to accept consulting jobs that took me away from the comforts of my home, and thus, the safety of my routine. This presented some anxiety at first about whether I'd need the bathroom when I left the house; so I looked to my journal for the answer. At that time, it showed I needed the bathroom most often in the morning. After about two hours upon awaking, I was clear for the entire day. So I adjusted my wake up time in order to have two hours before leaving the house for work. This gave me confidence for the hectic and confined car ride to work, and left me enough time to prepare my lunch and snacks. My confidence even got a boost from working among the masses again because I was feeling better than I had in years. Best of all, I could work and stay on my road to recovery.

Avoiding Anxiety - Plan to Succeed

Planning was really the key word when I started venturing outside the house more often. It's a natural fact that I was going to have to deal with; I was feeling better and I wanted to get out. In the same way I got used to ordering when I was out at restaurants, I had to get used to thinking about my day: namely, what pills I'd need, and what kinds of food choices to bring. Eating out everyday wasn't the best idea on my program. I actually preferred the taste of my cooking, and it offered an extra zone of comfort for never having to worry about any non-diet ingredients getting in my food. This was no small bit of confidence to have, as we all know, stress of any kind is an energy drain, and a threat to our progress.

Snacks played a big roll in keeping me from getting weak, cranky, or unable to concentrate before each meal. I established my eating schedule in the first few months on the diet, and I wanted to stick to it because it was working. There's no telling when I was going to need a snack, or when that hunger would hit me, and I might not be around any good choices for safe food. *It didn't take long for me to realize that it was much better to have a snack and not need it, than to need it and not have it.*

It was always good for me to bring apples, a couple boxes of raisins, very ripe bananas, and other quick-grab fruit in my lunch bag. These were nutritious, super portable, and good to bring into long meetings. Keeping a couple of my cookies with me in a plastic bag proved, more times then not, to be a lifesaver. My nut mix (see Part 8, Favorite Recipes) was also a favorite in the car, or in-between meals at my office desk. I got caught many times standing in long lines at the registry of motor vehicles, or other public places, and that little bag of nut mix in my pocket saved the day. Learning to plan was the difference between being happy about my program, versus resenting that I couldn't run into a drug store for a candy bar when I was hungry. By planning ahead I avoided those potential traps and stayed on the road to success.

Obviously, anyone with IBD or IBS can be much more susceptible to anxiety than those without. My head felt like the same ol' me, but my body wasn't always cooperating. When I didn't listen to my body and I pushed it too far, I'd get out of my comfort zone. It would cause added stress, and often times frustrated feelings about my condition, even though I was healing and doing well on my program. Part of me would get impatient and want to be healed immediately, and it almost always happened when I got overtired. This was unnecessary suffering that could've been avoided.

With practice, I soon learned to reduce my anxiety by listening to my body, and getting what I needed when (or before) I needed it, primarily, food and rest. When I was tired, I'd go home and rest. It was that simple. I had to remember that while I felt "normal" and might have wanted to stay out late, it was because I was taking care of my body and staying on my program that I was even feeling that good to begin with. I had to respect my healing, go home, and get the rest I needed to keep on making progress. My logic was, by healing I'd be able to spend more quality time out as the months went on. And that's what I really wanted. Simple planning was the critical difference between enjoyable days, and stressful ones.

PART 4: The Ten Keys to My Success

As you could imagine, during eight years of searching I endured many challenges of mind, body, and of course, spirit. As if this nasty illness wasn't enough, my spirit was further challenged with other personal losses: a painful breakdown in my marriage, an eventual divorce, and a sudden economic downturn that claimed my business. Huge problems for anyone, let alone someone who's very sick. Add to it my desperate struggle for health with no map to follow, and I was definitely at a severe low point.

My ascent began when I realized that the onus was on me to change. No one else could do it for me. That's when I created this list. I knew I had a reason to persevere, but when times got dark with physical and emotional pain, it was easy to lose my spirit. I created these ten keys to keep me focused on my goal, elevate my spirit, and above all, inspire me to always persevere even in the face of defeat. These ten keys were forged during my battle and still work for me today in all areas of my life. Surprisingly, they also paved the way for a more confident, positive outlook that has changed my whole being.

STEVE'S 10 KEYS TO SUCCESS

1) Nothing is More Important Than Being Well
2) You are Stronger Than You Know
3) Discipline is a Friend
4) Come to Your Senses
5) Eat to Live, Don't Live to Eat
6) Be Good to Yourself
7) Listen to Your Body
8) Welcome Change
9) Be a Victor, Not a Victim
10) Get Rest

1) Nothing is More Important Than Being Well

This key is number one for a reason. No matter how down I got, I would remember this first key, and I'd be able to get up again. This is where I got my "fight." It was the key that saved me early on whenever I'd feel the temptation to cheat on the diet. I'd think about my health and how I could feel myself getting better. I'd think about how those good feelings just weren't possible when I was eating everything. "I deserve to be well," I'd say to myself, "I am not going to let anything stand in the way of my goal." I knew that my increased freedom to be outside, or do more normal tasks besides sit on a toilet, was way more important than the temporary sugar rush I'd get from a chocolate chip cookie. Nothing is more important than being well.

Every time I say this key to myself I feel stronger. It fuels my determination and makes my discipline not a chore, but a gift I can give to myself. It echoes the whole reason I started this quest to recover, and it keeps me on track. When I stay focused on my road to healing, I not only reap the rewards of increased freedom, I also gain greater self-respect. Think of this as a physical and spiritual 401K plan; now that's what I'd call investing in you.

2) You Are Stronger Than You Know

This motto is one of the best pieces of advice my grandma ever gave me. It was crucial to my success. At the time, I was so physically sick and mentally worn down that I didn't think I was capable of getting out of the bathroom, let alone having the ability to heal myself. But I had much to learn. My denial about my illness was beginning to break down. I could no longer lie to myself; I was sick and not getting any better with the medications available. I couldn't stand seeing myself as a physical and mental wreck anymore.

All I had to do to start was to believe. By believing I could help myself, I started the action necessary to move forward (i.e., begin a new diet and discover a program that worked for me). My early impatient attitude gave way to an understanding that many baby steps can equal giant leaps over time.

I have met many people that could easily identify how someone else needed to improve, yet they could not see how to improve themselves. For some it was denial that they even had a problem, and for others, maybe they never thought they could change. Just allowing themselves to even think of change might seem impossible. I believe challenging maybe, but definitely not impossible.

Human beings love comfort! We even like routines and patterns because they too are a form of comfort. Yet there are many patterns that are just not good for us, and deep down, we know it. (Is it any surprise that we also call comfort food, junk food?) Trouble is, it's hard to see patterns once you are in them. Yet, when I thought, "I am stronger than I know," it allowed me to look within myself and my lifestyle, and suddenly, the bad patterns became visible. For me, seeking them out and eliminating them from my life was well worth the effort. I have had the privilege of surprising myself and growing in mind, body and spirit. Once I saw what I had accomplished with this powerful concept I felt as if nothing could hold me back.

Belief in myself now affects all areas of my life. I don't say, "I can't" anymore. I don't see roadblocks anymore. That started by believing I could change, and then taking one step in the right direction. I didn't have to know exactly where I was headed, I just had to believe that I could help myself. When I believe I am stronger than I know, change *is* possible.

3) Discipline is a Friend

A friend of mine who once fell on hard times said, "You'd be amazed at what you can do without." I'd say that's a profound message. At first, discipline feels like we're depriving ourselves. And depending on how you're eating, in some ways, it is. But I too was amazed at what I could do without.

Like most of us, I cringed when I thought of the word discipline. For a long time, I used to think that discipline was my enemy; it's got such ugly connotations of pain and suffering, doesn't it? Like a high school football team running around a quarter mile track twelve times in all their gear. Such acts of discipline can appear to be exhausting and even pointless (especially when I was in high school). But oh how wrong I was. Making discipline my friend was the big mindset change I needed to help me succeed on my program. I like to say that it's the ugliest word you'll ever love. For me, it transformed my mindset of failure into a mindset of success.

The proof was in my journal. During my first attempt on the diet, all I could think about was what I was missing by being deprived of my favorite food. That mindset was just failure waiting to happen. I succeeded in my second attempt because I always thought about what I was gaining. I finally didn't care if I had another chocolate chip cookie for the rest of my life; that's when I knew I wanted to be well again more than anything else. I got it clear in my mind: by being disciplined and staying away from that kind of food, I was getting better. Discipline became my friend because I now could see what it gave me in return. That made staying on the diet infinitely easier. I never felt deprived again.

When I practice discipline, I remember that I'm also gaining another invaluable ally, patience. The two of these together make it easier to enjoy today on my program while I prepared for tomorrow. It fueled my determination in the beginning to make my motto: the easier I am on myself, the harder my life will be. As in, if I eat non-SCD™ food, I'll never be rid of this pain. I liked how that idea made me want to fight harder for my health, keeping me focused on healing. I could also apply this motto to everything in my life, from staying on my diet, to procrastinating about a project that I wish I'd just finish. So long as I didn't over do it, this motto really kept me going. The more I experience, the more it seems true.

When I was first diagnosed almost twenty years ago, I wanted the easy way to change - to take a magic pill and have all my problems disappear. But the waiting game always has you at someone else's pace. With discipline, I ensure that I am in control. Discipline puts me in the driver's seat. I'm not sitting on the sidelines waiting; I am active, doing everything I can to get in the game and live a more full life now. Twelve years of my life passed by while waiting for a magic pill; I wish I had those years back.

Without discipline, I wouldn't have made it to the state I'm in now. I wouldn't have the freedom I have now. I know I'd still be sick and miserable like I was. In hindsight, discipline was the easiest thing I could do to help myself. Another way to say it might be, "There's nothing to it, but to do it." I respect it now for everything I've gained from it. Combined with determination, my discipline was unstoppable, and so was my eventual progress. Here's a journal entry from a bad day I had two months into Trial #6:

Even on a down day, I'm happy because I know I've got this program I can count on. It protects me. It's my shield against more pain, depression and hopelessness. I feel a comfort from my program... from the discipline. I've never felt that before. I never knew the peace that discipline could bring. I'm focused like a soldier, and this mission starts with me saving myself.

4) Come to Your Senses

Using my senses is a wonderful gift to give to myself. It has a calming and peaceful effect that centers me, and naturally generates good feelings. This keeps me from getting caught up in the natural noise of the mind (e.g., always seeking control, feeling pressure of the day, hurried, etc.), which can be a vicious trap of negative feelings for us all, and even worse for those of us with gut illness. During my trials, I discovered that *the senses are my best defenses.* It's easy to remember, and it's something we all have. Why not use it to our advantage?

For example, when the sunlight shines in on me through a window, or while I'm outside, I take a moment to feel its warmth on my face and just acknowledge how good it feels. Or when I'm working at the computer, I like to tune into the feeling of my fingers against the keys while I type the words. It's as simple as that. I just make time throughout the day to pay attention to my senses. It becomes a thrill to just witness these simple things. I began to see that every waking minute allowed me the opportunity to collect positive reinforcement from my senses, all just from tuning in. When I saw how peaceful and grateful it made me feel, I thought what a shame it is to take them for granted. When I remember to recognize them, I tap into all the powerful joy my life can afford me.

By using my senses I avoid getting sucked up into my mind's traps of self-pity, even while in a flare-up! It helps me to not focus on the moments of physical pain, or allow them to become the definition of my whole experience. It helps me to not lose sight of all the other things my body does well. And in reality, those far outweigh the fact that I have been "digestively challenged." No longer did I think of myself as "doomed" or "chronically ill." This was a massive shift in my outlook on life - from the glass half empty, to the glass half full. No pill has ever done that for me. Cultivating these feelings of gratefulness from my senses was critical in helping me overcome the anger I had about my body. When I use my senses, I am happy just as things are. I am grateful for all the things I can do. I am grateful for all the joy I can feel. And it only gets better as I heal on my program.

5) Eat to Live, Don't Live to Eat

I love that simple phrase. I first thought of it not too long after I started my program. Before trying the SCD™, I was living at the mercy of my taste buds; I ate what I craved all the time. If you're like me, admitting that you're a slave to your cravings didn't come easy, but as they say, "That's when the healing begins!" It was obvious right away that the diet is healthy; no longer could I just binge on crackers and cookies, I was now going to eat a balanced variety of the healthy foods. Substitutions were made. Raisins became my chocolate chips. Honey became my sugar. Almond flour became my bread.

Traumatic taste-bud modification you might think? Hardly. I knew everything I was eating was actually good for me for a change and would now help me heal instead of hurt me. That softened any pain from feeling deprived. I learned quickly from this time that cheating on the diet is not a reward. To be successful on the diet, I had to replace the way I thought about celebrating or comforting my ups and downs. Food should no longer be the go-to remedy. And once I really understood that, I was free. It was the key that made it so much easier to stay on the diet. For the first time in my life, I felt in control. Not only did my guts feel better almost immediately, you could see it in my face with healthy skin. So when I'd get those familiar crunchy, munchy, hunger-pangs, I made up a slogan that always saved me: *I will not eat anything that doesn't help my body.*

Clearly, the diet opened my eyes: food can be medicine, or food can be poison. Food can help me, or food can hurt me. Do you really need a nutritionist to tell you that eating cookies for breakfast, lunch, and dinner is not good for you? Yet, there are those of us who do. I did, but I finally came around to wanting to play a bigger role in helping myself be healthy. Soon I understood that *food is really just fuel.* You wouldn't try to run your car on dirt, would you? You need the right fuel! Your body does too. It's important for everyone, and even more important for us as we try to improve our health.

It helped my transition to eating healthy by remembering that food is also an industry. And all those food networks, chefs, and processed food companies benefit financially by making food become an obsession. Those are some heavy forces against us. But without all their noise and profit driven agendas, food is really just fuel. So to keep me well and committed to the diet, that became my new mantra.

It's not that the SCD™ is unappetizing or unexciting, actually, the diet has substitutes for everyone. Have you ever seen a person overdose on nectarines? It just doesn't happen. The diet changed my state from poor nutrition, to getting all my nutrients in a day and enjoying it. I also found that almond flour makes very flavorful and extremely nutritious breads, baked goods, pizza and more. Best of all, almond flour left me satisfied. Unlike wheat flours, I didn't get those mad cravings to fill up on it at the exclusion of fruits and vegetables. This was a major milestone, one that will have a positive effect on me for the rest of my life.

I went from thinking about and eating snack food all the time, to being able to walk down the junk food aisle at the grocery store and not even notice it. It took me a couple months to really own that mindset, but it was worth the effort for one of the most liberating feelings I ever had in my life. I can easily say that going on the diet was one of the best decisions I ever made. Life is too short to be "chained" to a toilet; I want to get out there and live it! And to do so, I eat to live.

6) Be Good to Yourself

No success is too small to make a big deal out of, especially while healing. I noticed that once I started feeling better on my program, I almost immediately began to get impatient. I wanted to be done with the program instantly; I wanted to be healed immediately, yesterday was too late. I became aware of this impatience and realized it was creating daily tension, making me more than a bit grumpy. And who likes grumpy people? So I knew I needed to change. I had to work with myself, not against myself, and that's when I learned that to do, I had to be good to myself. When we are feeling good, it's easy to take our health for granted. It seems that as modern life gets more hectic, people tend to take care of themselves less and less. That's not good for anyone, especially for those with gut illness. Intestinal disease is a breeding ground for exhaustion, and learning to give myself a break was a big advancement in making my life and my healing easier.

In the beginning of healing, it took me a while to accept that certain tasks are just going to take me more time. No one wants to see themselves as sick, but putting extra pressure on your already sick body only makes things worse. This is a big mistake and part of the inherent denial I found associated with this illness. I was guilty of over-tasking, trying to make up for that time I lost on the toilet, to the point where I'd be exhausted. Then I'd really lose time because I needed to rest from being exhausted. I found it's much better to accept my present condition and temporarily say, "Today I'll get only half of this job done, then tomorrow I'll continue or finish the job depending on how much energy I have." It's more important to respect your body while healing and cut everything you do in half. Though it might take me longer to finish, I found that the sense of accomplishment in completing realistic goals (half the job, quarter of the job, etc.) was far more beneficial for my well-being. Remember, many baby steps make giant leaps.

I was also good to myself by not abusing my body like I used to. When I found myself eating in a hurry, I'd slow down, take smaller bites of food, and chew them carefully and mindfully. The goal was to focus on my body's actions and the real flavor of the food. This was working with myself. This was not only helping my body work less during digestion, but it was far more relaxing to take time out to enjoy my food. Just to simply take your time eating. These little hidden moments can provide opportunities for feelings of joy. Your day is full of them, tune in and make yourself happier.

Another way I was good to myself was by not playing a waiting game with my healing. While healing the first time through, I found myself judging every bathroom visit I had, hoping that with each day some miraculous change was going to unveil itself. Sure, it was a natural reaction, but it made for a lot of extra tension to carry. The second time through on the diet was even worse because I remembered how good I felt the first time, and how I couldn't wait to get back there. The third time through, I was grateful to even be healing at all, and that felt like a much better way to be. So it pays to see the big picture; it makes a big difference. I did my daily bathroom business no matter if it was one, two, or three times, and I forgot about it after I left the bathroom. I put the emphasis on the life I was living and on the activities I could now do, instead of the other things I hoped to be doing soon. I saw my progress over weeks or a month. It made me feel gifted rather than frustrated – and there's a big difference between living a day with either of those feelings, it affects the whole day.

You can't live in the past or the future. When you try, it denies you the joy of the present. The present moment is all I have. I am being good to myself when I remember that in the present moment, I have everything I need. I thought a little reworking of the famous John Lennon quote was good to remember while on my program: life is what happens while you're waiting to heal.

7) Listen to Your Body

Every *body* is different. My success was due in large part to my ability to listen to my body. Like a scientist, in my trials I would try a new variable and record what happened. I had to listen to my body in order to make the necessary changes in my program to progress, and eventually heal. Without listening, there would have been no progress. I had to work on observing, but with practice I improved quickly.

There are treatments that doctors suggest which work for some people, but not for others. There are foods on the SCD™ that might not give some people trouble, but did for me. By listening, I learned how my body reacted to something I ate; it also helped me understand when I was just having another brief Herxheimer reaction from the probiotics in my program. Learning to listen to your body is the same kind of intuition that you use when you are sick with a cold. It's that simple: take care of yourself! By listening to my body, I could adjust the diet to help myself. For example, when I was in a flare-up or Herxheimer reaction, I'd look to cutting back on my raw fruit, nuts, and raw vegetable intake.

Keeping a daily journal just makes sense while on a program for growth. It was also instrumental in helping me listen to my body. Seeing positive change in my journal brought about even more feelings of accomplishment and happiness. It was hard to argue with the data. Just as important, it serves as a place to go back to if your gut isn't feeling good and you need to track down any changes that might have occurred in diet, supplements, or medications. My food journals definitely made it easier for me to track that peanut butter reaction I had.

I also loved keeping a personal journal for my thoughts and feelings. This was another type of listening to my body that was both fun and beneficial. I wrote down whatever I wanted, even if it was totally unrelated to the healing program I was on. It was a nice break. It also allowed for validation of my voice and spirit, which kept my interests and thoughts alive and growing in a positive direction.

8) Welcome Change

When I first embarked on the SCD™ in 1998, it was challenging for me. Let's face it; change is hard for everyone, mostly because we fear the unknown. It's easy to understand; you don't know what the new thing is or how it works, so you fear the worst. I've seen it in myself. But if you think about all the things you can do, like drive a car, or play a sport, weren't they also once uncomfortable because you didn't know how to do them yet? Bet you can't think of your life without them now. How sad it would be.

The diet taught me that the strange feelings of change signify that growth is starting. Like how awkward your hands might feel on the guitar at your first lesson. While these awkward feelings are natural, it helps to remember they are just temporary. What makes me happy when I feel these growing pains is just that I feel them. It's the signal that I am growing and changing – that itself becomes a reward. What fun is it to stay the same all through life? How boring! Especially when there is so much you can do to help yourself by learning like I did with my program.

There is fun in change when you become aware of it and welcome it. There is joy to be had in not knowing exactly where you are going, but feeling good about the direction. It makes life feel like an adventure, always learning something. And to me, that's a wonderful way to live. I think of it as, if you face your fear, you automatically choose to trust yourself. And that is a powerful ally. History has countless examples of people who welcomed change and discovered incredible things. Would rock and roll sound very different today if a guy named Chuck Berry didn't believe in himself and his style? You bet it would.

Finding a new hobby, or delving into an interest that you never had time for is a great way to welcome change. You get to learn more about this world and yourself at the same time. Plus, it's a fun way to pass the time while healing.

9) Be a Victor, Not a Victim

There was a time when I was practically a recluse (imagine Howard Hughes without all the money). This illness can do it to you, and it took me a while to even realize it. Every time we'd go out, it seemed as if I was always telling my wife, "Honey, I think we need to go home, I'm not feeling good again." It was real pain, embarrassment, and of course, frustration. And that was while I was on my prescribed medication. For me, I couldn't just sit around and wait anymore for drug companies to come up with a cure while my life was wasting away in agoraphobia-land. I once had a doctor tell me, "They'll cure this illness in your lifetime." That was 1989. Now, they're still offering the same pills for my illness, and there still is no cure. How much more of my life was I going to spend inside waiting? The fact is, if I didn't start looking for ways to heal myself other than just medication, I'd still be that sad victim confined to the bathroom, a prisoner in my own house.

When I'm not feeling good, I'm the one who's missing out. The rest of the world doesn't stop for me. How much is missing out on one year of my life worth? Now multiply that by how many years I've been ruled by the illness. (You can see where this is headed.) I had my answer. *I'm the only one who hurts when I don't try to help myself.* I had to try.

What it took was a step in the right direction. The day I made my first step not to take it anymore was the day I became a victor and left being a victim behind. That's what I needed, a real today-is-the-first-day-of-the-rest-of-my-life attitude. I like it because it's good for lots of issues, health related and otherwise, that seem to bring us down. The victim mentality is so wrong for so many reasons, worst of which, it doesn't help us! Hey, it goes without saying that all of us would rather be bald, or fat, or whatever than have gut illness, but that's life. Some things we can't choose.

What we can choose is if we want to sit around playing the victim and continue being sick, or stand up, be a victor, and fight for a chance to heal.

It reminds me of a time from my first trial. I was sitting in my favorite breakfast diner one day struggling with the diet. Constantly I felt on the outside of life, ordering my two scrambled eggs with burnt bacon when I really wanted old fashioned pancakes with syrup! It seemed like there was no way out. When I ate foods off the diet, my symptoms got worse. When I stuck to the diet, I felt like I was missing something. Actually, I was, but it wasn't pancakes and syrup.

I paid my bill and sadly walked past all the other "normal" people who appeared to be eating anything they wanted. I was late for a contractor at my house, so I rushed home and forgot about my woes for the time. The contractor finished his job expertly, but as he left he seemed sad, like something was bugging him inside. I knew that look well, so we started talking and sure enough, he was sad. All the money and success he had couldn't find him the perfect wife. He just turned thirty and already he was starting to give up. I felt his pain as he recounted his story. Suddenly, I understood that we were both playing the victim instead of realizing that we were lucky: we could do something about our conditions.

We can only help ourselves, and sitting around moping and playing the victim wasn't helping me. It was hurting me. I was putting my life on hold; I had stopped living. I didn't want to be like that. Right then and there I chose to see myself as lucky in this fight against gut illness. There are many diseases I know of where putting up a fight is barely an option. I counted my blessings; it was time to be a victor not a victim. Family and loved ones benefit too, and don't be surprised if they notice the "old you" is back.

The feeling of finally regaining my health is one of the greatest of my life; it's a gift that keeps on giving. That's a massive reward that reminds me of what a simple step in the right direction can bring. It's a lesson that I can't forget. It took me four years of my life to learn this lesson. I hope that none of you waste that much of your precious time.

10) Get Rest

Chronic illness is an enormous strain on a person. When we're not on the toilet, we might feel like we have to play "catch up" for our lost time, and that can be exhausting. Fighting back for my health took energy too, and therefore I needed more rest. There are more and more studies in which researchers are starting to point to lack of sleep for feelings of depression, irritability, and more. Clearly, this is a threat to the positive attitude I needed for my program. Exhaustion can cloud judgment, make you feel agitated, irritable or just hopeless – even when that isn't the reality. This happened to me several times early on when I was very sick. My confidence was so low that I almost didn't want to continue with my program.

Rest was critical to give me the positive attitude to continue. No one can make a wise decision when exhausted; everyone needs rest. Meditation and mind games help, but they don't take the place of good ol' fashioned sleep. The best cure I've found when I'm feeling those overtired blues is to just admit that I'm tired, don't say much else, and go get rest. On overtired days, I try to go to bed early so I can wake up feeling positive, and ready to keep healing.

The stages of my recovery proved how important the intestines are to feelings of overall well-being. Before starting out on my program, I was tired all the time because my intestines were not functioning properly, leaving me often exhausted and cranky. As my program brought me results, I noticed an increase in positive energy, and a decrease in feeling tired and grumpy. I learned to take time out in my early stages of healing to get rest. It was an easy way I could help the healing, and a smart move to keep me on the path for success.

PART 5: How I Overcame the Roadblocks

To me, this section is one of the most important in the book. It would've saved me a lot of frustration and heartache if I had it back in 1998 when I started my trials. This section is all about how I beat the roadblocks I came across during my journey. What follows is my first hand experience with these issues, and the solutions I created to help me stay happier, and focused on my path to success. I hope this insight can serve and inspire others as a reference for a smoother journey.

Roadblock: I Don't Think I Can Do the Diet

Breakthrough: I am capable of far more than I allow myself to believe.

It was spring 1998. I was in a prolonged flare-up, needing the toilet an average of twenty times a day. I was also indulging my cravings in bad food choices. I had just finished reading about the SCD™, and while the concept of ridding my body of IBD was tempting, I was also strongly compelled not to do anything for fear that abstaining from junk food might just kill me. Hilarious as it seems, the concept of living without it had never occurred to me before.

Back then, I drank a six-pack of cola a day on average, and seriously wondered how I was going to change my ways when I couldn't go an hour without a candy, soda, or some kind of bread-cracker-pretzel-snack food. It's an interesting aspect of human nature to ponder: as desperate as I was to be well, I hesitated when I first learned of a diet change to help myself. I guess deep down I was afraid that depravation and discipline were synonymous with pain and more pain, and I was already living in lots of that. Also disconcerting was that in Elaine's book on the SCD™, she made no guarantees that the diet worked for everyone. If I tried it, I would be depriving myself and still may not get the desired result. Think of all those sugar rushes I'd be missing out on! Oh, how awful!

But running out of options other than surgery, I decided to forge ahead. As you can read in my first trial, I had about a fifty percent reduction in bathroom trips. I stayed on it for almost two years, and though I was disappointed that the diet didn't heal me on its own, I couldn't help but be amazed that I actually made it so long without junk food. So even though I was striving for one goal and missed, I completely succeeded at another that I wasn't even trying for. As a result, I proved to myself that I was strong enough to change, and that was the most important milestone of my life. It was also the discovery I needed to motivate me as I continued to search for my solution.

Even though change isn't easy for most of us, I found it comforting to remember that growth is not possible without it. When the discomfort of change comes, I remind myself that it's natural and expected. To me, it's a good sign that transition (i.e., growth) is looming.

I became a believer that huge progress can be started with just one baby step. When I was tired and beaten physically and emotionally, that baby step was all I could muster. But it was also all I needed. It was true, I was afraid of the unknown, most of us are. But what made my escape possible was that I did not want to be ruled by that fear anymore. And that small effort paid off with huge rewards when I discovered I was capable of far more than I was allowing myself to believe. For me, it's a lesson that's hard to forget: *I am stronger than I know*. Even now when I hesitate and think I can't complete a daunting new task, that lesson continues to motivate me to take that first step. You definitely wouldn't have this book in your hands without it.

Roadblock: Cravings, Temptations and Feeling Deprived

Breakthrough: No food tastes as good as freedom feels.

I'm convinced that my ability to stay with the diet on my second attempt was no accident. My breakthrough began from a simple realization: I was eating food to make myself happy.

The first time I tried the diet, I definitely had days of feeling deprived. It's just natural. But what made sticking to the diet easier the second time was realizing that certain foods (i.e., those not on the SCD™) were actually hurting me. Elaine Gottschall spent years proving this (the subject of her book, *Breaking the Vicious Cycle*) and if that wasn't enough, I could always rely on my own proof: taking the bread and sugar out of my diet cut my bathroom trips in half! My first trial proved it, and I most certainly appreciated not having to go to the bathroom twenty times a day. Ten times, while still a lot, was definitely much better. Of course, there was always the pain; that was easy to remember. The foods the diet omits (especially all my old snack favorites) made my stomach hurt, and I'm especially not fond of that nasty gut pain.

It became clear to me that eating food my digestive system could not process stood in the way of my healing. And that made me angry. I didn't want anything to stop me from getting this wretched illness out of my body, especially if I had a say in it. And just like that, the line was drawn. What was once my friend, now became my enemy. What once tasted good, now tasted like poison. I couldn't even bring it to my lips anymore when I thought about what it was doing to me. And that's when I knew I had made a breakthrough. I started saying that, "No food tastes as good as freedom feels," and I no longer felt deprived.

As I began to denounce all my former cravings and temptations, I also began to feel special, almost super human. It was fantastic! Almost overnight, I could walk down any food store candy aisle, the same one that had stopped me so many times before, and for the first time, just laugh. I felt it in my walk. I felt it in my smile. I knew I was now truly "the boss of me." It was one of the greatest feelings I had ever felt.

Roadblock: Feeling Sorry for Myself / Why Me?

Breakthrough: Focus on what I can do, not what I can't.

This was a tough one when I first started my program, but that's what really made me search hard for the breakthrough. In the beginning, I was filled with those "Why me" thoughts: why did I have to go through this extra daily effort? What did I ever do to deserve this awful illness? And of all things, did it have to be a pooping problem? After a while I realized that I was stuck being miserable waiting for answers to these questions when really, there were no answers. And as long as I kept waiting, I'd remain stuck in a sad place.

This is what makes self-pity so dangerous, it is immobilizing! We all have a reason at some time or another to fall into this trap. The "Why Me" question is a natural one at first; it is a human response to a shock. But gone unchecked, it can quickly turn into a victim mindset, a difficult trap to escape because it's often hard to see that you're in it. That's why I created three philosophies for myself to keep the "Why me" blues away.

First: struggling with my own illness gave me a new view into the struggle of others, people with all kinds of illnesses. The benefit of this was great; it increased my awareness and compassion for everyone who struggles with physical limitations and in doing so, I recognized my own strength. My experience has shown me that people with physical challenges often have the potential to grow far beyond a person without. I'm constantly amazed when I recognize how little belief people can have in themselves. And it doesn't surprise me either that most of those people have no physical limitations.

Second: don't think you're lucky? Sure, I may have been handicapped when I needed a bathroom twenty times a day, but it's what I call invisibly handicapped. I don't need a wheelchair, or a cane; I can hide it if I want to. (Although, it does get harder when you get over ten times a day!) There are many handicapped people who are not so lucky, and we have to remember that at least we have a chance to relieve our situation, and that shouldn't be taken for granted. In essence, that's what The Gut Help™ Program is: a chance to escape this condition.

Years ago, when I was in high school, a fellow neighbor and classmate lost his battle with cancer. It was so tragic and horrible to realize that someone could die so young, especially a friend. When I visit my hometown and drive by his former house, my problems seem very small, and my blessings seem great. I know that if he was alive today, I'm sure not much would bother him, and life would seem beautiful just to be here. That's the big picture we can't forget. When I think of him, it reminds me that even though IBD and IBS also remain a mystery to the medical world, at least I had a chance to escape. And as difficult as my illness was, now you know why I think I'm very lucky. Even though I had to fight hard for years to find my program, I am grateful every day that I even had a chance to take.

Third: And if none of these philosophies worked for me, there was always the famous quote from Charles Bukowski, "Self-pity is the most useless of all emotions." I'd have to say that I couldn't agree more. I was guilty of being so trapped by self-pity early on that I know I became a burden to my wife and family. Who would want to be around someone like that? Someone who is always down, even when there's a chance to be well. Of course my family hated seeing me sick, but I had to be the one to stop my knee-jerk, self-pity reaction, if for no other reason than for them. I did it by quickly recognizing those feelings of self-pity when I felt them coming on, and I'd fight back by emphasizing what I can do, not what I can't. It made me positive instead of negative. I wasn't going to let this illness or the challenges of my program stop me from the positive role I had had in my family before. If I have one regret, it's that I didn't put a stop to my self-pity sooner.

Roadblock: Feeling Alone / Isolated

Breakthrough: Focus on the time I'm having, not the food.

Journal entry from three months into Trial #6:

Even though there's much to celebrate being on my program, I think it's totally normal to sometimes get discouraged at this early stage. For instance, I was at a wedding reception this past weekend, and at my table I was the only one not eating bread. As positive as I was that day, I felt alone and left out. Even though I knew that the bread would make me sick if I ate it, I just didn't want to feel different.

But is being different so bad? Where would I be if I weren't on my program? That was an easy question to answer: I certainly wouldn't be at that wedding reception, that's for sure! I wouldn't be able to go because I'd be home running to the bathroom twenty times a day. And that's what being alone and isolated really feels like. It's the kind of "different" I didn't want to be anymore. Because healing isn't instantaneous,

I have to remind myself that I'm always improving as long as I stay true to my program. My breakthrough came when I focused on the time I was having, not the food. I was glad to be part of this party, and that was much more important than eating any bread.

And who's to say that there weren't others at that table with IBD or IBS? They might still be in denial, or just didn't know that they could do something to help themselves. The reality is that most people do suffer with some type of illness in their lives, and there is no magic pill for many of those illnesses. Start talking with others and you'll see that we are not alone in our struggle. You may also be surprised at who admits they have your illness, which can make your friendship even better, or introduce you to a new best friend.

Being on my diet can also make you feel special in a good way. It did for me. It was like I had a secret that was saving me. I was on a mission, and as long as I stayed true to it, I got results. I also noticed that staying away from all the junk food traps when I was out, often gave me a feeling of power. Many times when a friend would see me eating one of my cookies I brought along in a bag, they'd ask to try it. They couldn't believe how good it tasted, so much better than junk food. All of a sudden, I was seen as the guy who knew good food. I have to admit, it's fun feeling like a secret, healthy revolutionary.

Ultimately, what made me feel best was that I knew I wasn't hurting my body when I ate. On my program I am finally getting better; it may not be instant, but it's always heading in the right direction. So if I ever feel that I'm alone, and this diet makes me feel different, I remember that I am reaching my goals, and that's the kind of different I don't mind being.

Roadblock: Getting Sick on Top of Being Sick (stomach flu)

Breakthrough: Make diet adjustments, and remember that by staying with my program, I'm helping myself get through it as fast as possible.

Journal entry from two months into Trial #7:

As I sit here with a nasty flu bug, I'm reminded that times like these are really the hardest. I feel trapped from all angles. The flu bug is wreaking havoc on my already challenged intestines, like adding fuel to the fire. Even the mellowest stomach flu can cause me added discomfort. I feel like I'll never get back to normal, even though I know this will pass. It's hard to take a painful set back like this, especially when I was getting excited with all the progress. So it's a downer that my pain and bathroom trips have increased, and that I now have to cut back on the raw fruits and veggies that I'm used to.

This recent stomach flu that was going around town was severe. My cramps were so bad that I could hardly stand. I had to resort to heavy Pepto Bismol for three days. It's going on a week with no signs of improving, and that's been tough, reminding me just how much I hate the kind of pain I feel. But that also reminds me of exactly why I'm on my program: I don't want to feel that pain anymore! And what gets me through times like these is to remember that a set back like this is normal, and will work its way out. I'm doing all I can do for myself by sticking with my program, there's no better way I know to help myself get over this flu faster.

My doctor once told me, "People with IBD and IBS take longer to get over a stomach flu. It's expected." During these times, I figured out that I could help myself by doing everything I know to ease my pain: namely, get my rest, and increase water consumption. I also stop probiotic increases temporarily. In this way, my body is able to get rid of the flu as fast as it can without having to also adjust to an increase in probiotics. In addition, I immediately put a hold on all raw fruits and veggies, replacing them with smaller portions of cooked veggies and applesauce until I feel better. This is a big pain saver. My wife was over the flu in two days, for me, it was more like seven. The challenge wasn't the flu so much, it was resisting impatience.

What gives me the most comfort is that my program feels like a shield. It protects me against the food that aggravates the illness, and feelings of hopelessness. My data shows that as long as I stay with it, I'm doing the most I can do for myself, working on a way out of pain instead of always being its prisoner. And during a flu, it's good to remember that by staying with my program, I'm helping myself get through it as fast as possible, and that's all that I could wish for.

Roadblock: Stressed Out

Breakthrough: Use my body to bring my mind gently back to equilibrium.

It's easy to see how gut illness can stress someone out. Worrying about finding a bathroom and if I could get there in time, was always a miserable and relentless stress for me. Even though the diet helped minimize that stress, it initially created a stress of its own. At first, it was a little freaky to walk into my usual grocery store, and see that I could no longer eat all the items they had on display. Then it got a little trickier when I began reading labels, and noticing that many items had some form of bad starch or sugar, which are not allowed on the diet. But soon those items became invisible to me, and I immediately gravitated to the foods I could have, which are healthy and plentiful. I just wasn't "seeing" them before.

I also needed time to get used to baking my own food. Whatever initial complaints I had were cast aside when my cookies and bread creations came out of the oven. They tasted so fresh and delicious, much better than anything I used to eat. And I really loved knowing that these treats wouldn't hurt my gut.

Still, the stress of the real world has a way of sneaking up on anybody. But with practice, I'm getting much better at noticing it when it does. Now I'm quick to catch any signs of increased irritability, or feelings like I can't keep up. To me, these are the warning signs that I'm getting stressed out. The great news is that the quicker I jump on them and start to de-stress, the quicker I feel better and keep stress from affecting my sensitive gut. That's why it's important to watch for signs of stress; we don't want anything to slow our progress. My doctor once told me that stress doesn't cause IBD or IBS, but it can aggravate it. This is yet another reason to have a plan in place for when I get those stressed out feelings.

The most powerful weapon I can use against stress is my body. When I used to get stressed out, I was unable to talk or think myself out of it. It was as if my brain just shut down, and couldn't see beyond the stress. So I tried another approach, and found much success by using my body to bring my mind gently back to equilibrium. Being physical was the key to calming my mind. Instead of letting the stress build up on me like it used to, I practice listening to my body to catch it before it hits those levels. When I notice that I'm getting stressed, I simply follow one or more of my favorite de-stress activities. The list that follows is was what works best for me.

Steve's 6 favorite ways out of stress:

1) *Prioritize to do lists.* Watch out for trying to get too much done in a day, it can cause loads of silent stress.

2) *Listen to my body signals.* Tune in. Learn to sleep when I'm tired, and watch for muscle twitches. For me, they are signals of exhaustion. I try not to postpone this request from my body, and take a nap if necessary.

3) *Yoga.* My favorite "instant" de-stressor. It works wonders for me because my focus is on my body and breath as I try to do the exercises correctly. I begin to unwind greatly, even at the initial breathing stages; that always amazes me. Taking time out to be aware of my body, as in Yoga, gets me out of my head, and creates a sublime feeling of peace that simply has no equal. Yoga feels like a meditation for my body. I enjoy its benefits throughout the rest of my day. It is difficult not to feel peaceful and grateful after even a short Yoga practice.

4) *Exercise.* Weight lifting or jogging always clears my head, but it's important not to push myself, or let the scheduling of these activities also become a stress. It is also wise not to begin any exercise program without consulting your doctor first. I waited six months on my program before I was ready for an increase in exercise intensity, and only after I spoke with my doctor. (See Part 3 for my exercise schedule and routines.)

5) *Try massage.* Every once in a while, a day spa with a relaxing setting does wonders for your time out of mind. Another benefit is that it is excellent for learning the art of mindfulness by focusing your attention on just your body in the moment. Sure, it can be expensive, but it's nice to treat yourself occasionally. You are definitely worth it.

6) *Morning meditation.* This helps immensely to carry-on the benefits of the previous activities. I find that early morning is the easiest time to be quite and peaceful. It is a perfect time to be grateful, practice mindfulness (the art of staying in the present moment), and slowly center myself before my work begins. I practice this every day, which goes a long way toward keeping me centered and de-stressed.

Roadblock: The Mindless Munching Habit

Breakthrough: Allow the diet to help me establish better eating habits.

Journal entry from one month into Trial #1:

Too many nuts the day before means lots of bathroom pain today! It draws glaring attention to my compulsive noshing habits of old. Noshing is a fun word for mindlessly munching, as in sit-in-front-of-the-TV-and-"inhale"-a-bag-of-pretzels.

My "big duh" realization today is that I shouldn't carry-over my old noshing habit to the SCD™, such as eating too many nuts in exchange for eating too many pretzels. It's a non-helpful behavior, and substituting it won't solve anything, it can actually cause pain. I've got to use this change in diet to also reprogram my portion control. It's time to finally get that under control. I've got to stop noshing altogether because it's just not good to eat too much of any one food. I must eat balanced; I can feel the diet works better like that, and I hurt less too! This is a gradual reprogramming process that I know I can master. I may eat too many nuts at one sitting, but at least I'm catching myself now. It's a healthy, fun challenge to practice.

I can see what this diet really is: it's the right way to eat. I realize that for me to be successful, I must completely reprogram my former eating habits. And it's time I do it. With gut illness, I can't do that mindless eating like I used to and not pay a price. Even people without gut illness "pay" for noshing by becoming obese, unhealthy, and prone to disease, all of which can keep them from reaching their goals.

The SCD™ is a great diet because it helps reprogram my old haphazard eating style. It gets me thinking about balanced meals, and that in turn helps promote portion control, and improved health. It curbs binging, which results in keeping my weight in check, as well as giving me optimal nutrition.

Roadblock: Diet Feels Like a Prison

Breakthrough: Don't miss out on what you can enjoy now.

Journal entry from six months into Trial #7:

It's important while I'm fighting the good fight on the SCD™ not to get so focused that I forget I'm living my life. That's an easy way to create a prison for myself. For example, I was working-out downstairs this morning, and I started thinking about cleaning up our workshop, or writing out a movie idea just for kicks. It was a nice escape from all my journaling, and food planning. It felt great to just change my way of thinking, from disciplined and organizational, to creative and freethinking. Like a breath of fresh air, it made me realize the value in taking time out for these activities. I recognize that they have an important place in my healing too.

I have found that working with my spirit, instead of criticizing it, really makes my life much more fun. That means following those creative impulses when I get them without judgement. This gives me a liberating feeling that's therapeutic because it frees my spirit as my program is freeing my body. Also, the diet just seems easier now than in the beginning. Time helps, most definitely.

I think of the diet as learning how to drive a car with a standard (manual shift) transmission - once you get it, you never forget it. At first I had to think about shifting, but after a while, it just became second nature; I was shifting to all the right gears instinctively. The diet became the same way for me. After a while, I began making the right choices automatically. That's a great moment. Whenever I felt like the diet was limiting, I made a real effort to refocus my attention on what I could eat, not what I couldn't. Remember, there's so much to enjoy right now! I helped myself by giving the foods on the diet a chance; if it weren't for this diet, I never would have known how good a ripe peach could taste!

Today, six months in, I don't see myself as hopeless and stuck like I used to. I see a way out. Since I am feeling much better, and I've got a handle on the diet, this might be a good time to take a break from writing down everything that I eat. I wouldn't stop recording my bathroom trips or sticking with the diet. But the extra free time I would gain gives me a boost of confidence to go out and enjoy the new lwvwl of freedom I've earned.

Roadblock: Impatience

Breakthrough: What might be considered slow progress is still progress nonetheless.

Journal entry from one month into Trial #9:

In the beginning stages it's important to remember that what might be considered slow progress is still progress nonetheless. It helps me to remember what it was like before my program - when there was no progress at all - now that was hopeless. I am certainly not hopeless anymore.

Being impatient is a natural response when trying to get well, ask anybody with a cold! When I catch myself being impatient now, I stop and take comfort in knowing that everyday on my program is at least a step in the right direction. I recognize that I'm doing all I can do, and that should make anyone feel great. It's worth celebrating. There really are many things to enjoy right now, and that always helped me with impatience. It also helps to remind myself that my milestones will come, just as the progress I've seen already. I'll take stock in that.

Roadblock: Controlled by Illness

Breakthrough: By staying in touch with my joy, I don't allow this illness to control me.

I did have times when I felt this illness dictated my every move, mostly when I was on the toilet all the time before my program. It was an awful, trapped, hopeless feeling that didn't get better until my program gave me hope. Yet, even on the road to healing there were still some rough days where I felt controlled by the illness.

During an early rough patch when I felt down, I stumbled on an idea one day. I would think of some fun things that I could do at the moment (hobbies, etc.) and just go do them, or at least one of them if I had only a short amount of time. The idea was to choose something that I hadn't had time for lately, and do it immediately. For me, it was almost always playing guitar. I could never spend enough time with it. It was always relaxing and quite the opposite of the other "have to" tasks I was routinely trapped by.

Sometimes, I preferred to just get outside and take a walk. Maybe take a different route, or sit on a park bench that I had always walked past and just stop to take in the moment. Other times I loved spending more quality time with my dog and playing fetch in a nearby park. I found it didn't take long to see the benefits of a short break (as little as fifteen minutes) so long as I was doing something fun that I missed doing. The point was to prove to myself that even this illness couldn't stop me from living my life fully. By staying in touch with my joy, I don't allow this illness to control me.

This short fun break (not food centered) would be just the right positive encouragement I needed when I felt controlled by the illness. It was like my own all-natural happy pill. It made me feel like I was really living my life now, instead of waiting for the day that I could live it. And that's what I really needed to feel. I loved it because it also seemed like taking revenge on this nasty illness. Some people say, "The best revenge is living well." And others, who like old Star Trek movies say, "Revenge is a dish best served cold." (I'm not sure I know exactly what that means, but Ricardo Montalban sure made it sound good.) *Either way, the point is that life is now; don't let it slip away while waiting for tomorrow.* Get into it today! Finally, I found a way to work with myself instead of against myself. And instead of always reaching for food to make me happy, I now had found a better way to be good to myself. When it worked like magic, I knew I was on to something.

I also helped myself in the beginning stages of my program by not thinking of myself as afflicted or different, even if I was rushing to find a bathroom. The important key here is not to dwell on it. I just did my thing, and moved right along. That was it. If I needed the bathroom more on one day, then I just needed the bathroom more on one day. As long as I was sticking to my program, I knew that my overall results were improving. My journals proved it, so I let that also be my inspiration.

Trying to laugh as much as possible was never a bad idea. It helped make me feel more normal, and less controlled by the illness. I'd often love to make fun of my situation, though it might seem a little odd, it actually proved to be hilarious at times. And I wouldn't disagree that there's still a lot of value in a well-timed toilet joke, especially for us. The power of laughter is mighty, and has dug me out of many a downer mood. I keep a well-stocked library of my favorite comedy movies, and I love seeking out new funny TV shows or stand-up comedians. Going out to movies with some of my friends who knew about my condition were also some great times. Being able to make jokes about my illness with them was a big release, and before I knew it, I'd be at a new level of health. Time flies when you're having fun, and it's really hard to feel controlled by an illness when you're laughing.

Roadblock: The Expected Early Flare-up on the Diet

Breakthrough: Review journals to see progress made up to this point. Remember how good being even a little better felt, and how it's worth it to stick it out to get back to that feeling again.

According to Elaine Gottschall's book, *Breaking the Vicious Cycle*, a flare-up in the second or third month into the SCD™ is not uncommon. I too experienced this in my trials on the diet. Although Elaine advised readers not to become discouraged, I found it impossible for me not to. I had been making excellent progress, and it's just natural that this roadblock would cause serious disappointment because it wasn't going away quickly.

I found this a particularly tough roadblock at first because it came so early on in the diet. After years of being a shut-in, I was finally improving and just starting to taste a little freedom. I was developing the right mindset and seeing the success of my new discipline, then… wham! I felt like I had lost it all. When the flare-up happened, my only thought was, "What was I doing wrong?" I hadn't forgotten Elaine's encouragement that it would pass; the reality was it still felt like a physical and emotional bummer. Within days, I went from partially formed stools to heavy diarrhea and cramps with increased bathroom trips necessary.

What made me not want to quit the diet was remembering the progress I had made up until this point. I reviewed my early positive journal entries. I thought about them.

I missed it. I had gotten a taste of freedom and health that I hadn't had in over a decade. I never knew how good even being a little better would feel until now. And I wanted it again, ASAP! It was worth it to me to stick it out during this challenging time, even if it wasn't going away as fast as a Herxheimer reaction would. I caught myself when I started to feel self-pity, and didn't allow it to snowball. Then I channeled my frustration into a more beneficial output: a deeper commitment to my diet. I began to think about all the outside activities I was going to do when I felt better because of staying with the diet, and that helped me pass the time positively.

I got over the flare-up in a little more than a week, and was back on track. Immediately, I did all the outside activities I had been thinking of. Talk about feeling grateful! It deepened my belief that when I stay on the diet, I am the one who benefits. It was an overwhelming confirmation that my freedom was definitely worth fighting for.

Roadblock: Food Allergies

Breakthrough: I use my journals to help track down any food allergies.

Every *body* is different. Just because the diet says a food is acceptable, it still may not be right for you. I found this out first hand, and I felt much better after I did, as it made way for faster improvements in my health. My method for finding my allergy was simple.

On a day that I would have excessive bathroom trips and heavy cramps (a.k.a. a bad toilet day), I would glance over the foods I ate to see if any stood out as common allergy culprits, like certain types of nuts (e.g., peanuts, cashews). If no common culprits appeared, then I'd just chalk it up as a Herxheimer reaction and leave it at that. If there were a common food culprit introduced, then I'd take a break from it, and try it again when I improved to see if had a similar reaction. Then, I used my journals to help review the last few days before the bad toilet day, and I tried to see if there was any new SCD™ food that I had added. I would mark the day in my journal as "BAD DAY" at the top of the entry, so it would be easy to cross-reference if I'd get a similar experience in the future. I also used this method when I was trying new foods that were SCD™ approved, but I had not eaten before.

This was how I discovered my peanut allergy. Peanuts and cashews actually have a huge amount of lactose in them, and often cause problems for people like me who are lactose intolerant. Before trying peanut butter I was feeling good, and was aware of my body's pattern of brief, occasional Herxheimer reaction days. I decided to cautiously add a few tablespoons of peanut butter to my diet every day, and soon found that I was regressing and my symptoms were increasing. These symptoms held on longer than my usual short Herxheimer reactions, and that's how I knew something had changed. Even though the diet allows peanuts after six months, after too many predictable bad toilet days with an excessive amount of cramps that I traced back to this culprit, I concluded that I was better off without them. When I stopped eating the peanut butter, my symptoms calmed down, and I again returned to making progress.

For me, I found it was best not to second-guess my Herxheimer reactions too much, especially in the beginning. It was one thing to be wary of common allergy culprits, and it's another to start ruling out foods that most likely would not cause an allergic reaction. I did this early on, and thought that my heavy Herxheimer reaction days were related to beef. I learned later, after many experiments of adding and removing beef, that I still had my Herxheimer reaction days regardless; they are part of the process. Keeping a good journal was instrumental in understanding my body's reactions, and adjusting the diet accordingly.

Roadblock: Flare-ups and Herxheimer reactions

Breakthrough: I don't dwell on an adjustment, and I celebrate when feeling good.

After quite a lot of experience, I learned the difference between my flare-ups and Herxheimer reactions. While both could have any combination of my old symptoms (repeated bathroom trips, cramps, convulsions, diarrhea and bleeding), it was the flare-ups that lasted longer. For me, the sign that I was in a flare-up would be the increases of any of my symptoms, especially blood with bowel movements, for at least a week. However, Herxheimer reaction days during my successful probiotic trials usually lasted only a day or two. That's a critical difference. So while they may feel the same, they most definitely are not. In a dramatic comparison, at my worst before my program, I was in a flare-up for almost a year. *My research shows that I experienced no flare-ups once I began taking certain probiotics (Trial #'s 7, 9 and 13).*

It helped me to think of my brief Herxheimer reactions as necessary adjustment days. Still, it's hard not to get down when one of these has your guts feeling taxed. Progress feels like it's stalled, even if it's temporary. When I'm having an adjustment day, it's easy to fall into the trap of dwelling on what isn't working. But I hit on a big positive boost when instead I started to look at what is working. I decided not to take it for granted, but to notice it. It was like my mind just jumped the sad ship, and got on board the happy one. I went from looking down to looking up. And I couldn't believe how quick I could make it happen, at times almost instantly.

The method I use is simple. I check-in with my gut; I pay attention to how it feels, and if I'm not in any pain at the moment, then I say to myself, "Hey! I'm feeling good!" I'd enjoy that feeling and be grateful. Soon I'd realize that the more I checked in with my body, I had more uptime than downtime, even during a few challenging adjustments. And that's all I needed to see. I try to leave that pain behind me in the bathroom when I close the door because I know that I'm on my way to making that pain less and less. I'd come out, rest for a bit, focus on the positive, and then get on with my day - no grumpy feelings or faces necessary. The key was that I didn't allow myself to get caught up in the minor discomfort of an adjustment. I realized that it's OK to need time to rest if I feel some pain, but when I feel good, then notice that I feel good. I was happy to not be hurting all the time and I wasn't going to take it for granted! That saved me by making any adjustment day fly by and showed me that I can still have a great time even when not feeling my best. It's important to note that usually no more than an hour or two after even the worst Herxheimer reaction, I always got back to feeling good. If I didn't, and the discomfort lasted longer or was unmanageable, I'd consider lowering my dosage of probiotics for that week until I was strong enough to continue.

The power of noticing is truly amazing. It can be tremendously useful to us all, especially those of us who are fighting to heal. During the initial stages of my program, it helped me stay happier by focusing on the beauty of being alive and not the sadness of being sick. I began to pay attention to simple things, like the uniqueness of a sneeze, or the music of washing my hands. It is staggering to notice these ordinary things and see them for what they really are: extraordinary. At times I would feel that I couldn't be as happy in the moment as someone who wasn't sick (or the quality of my life was such that it kept me from being happy), but I was wrong. I discovered that when I'm angry with my body, I'm the only person who loses; I lose out on being present for this amazing gift of life. I have the potential to do what others without illness often don't do: to be thankful for this moment, for the times I am feeling good. This keeps me peaceful and happy while I heal. It keeps me from waking up everyday with impatient thoughts of disappointment that I'm not fully recovered yet, because in the end those thoughts only rob me of this great moment I can live right now. And that would be a shame, because this moment is really all I have.

I developed a simple method that served me well in dealing with a flare-up, or adjustment day. First, I took care of myself physically and went into what I call "extra care mode." If I were exhausted from a heavy adjustment, I'd reschedule whatever appointments I had that day, and just rest until I felt better. I would adopt a temporary strict policy of no alcohol, nuts, raw fruit or raw veggies until the adjustment subsides. I would stick with just cooked veggies, very ripe bananas, and applesauce for my veggies and fruits until I felt better. I would still have my almond flour cookies, but I'd make sure not to go over four per day. I would also pay attention that I'm eating balanced meals (not too much of any one food – a good idea always), continuing to mind portion control (overeating is never good), and chew my food extra carefully, no gulping.

The key for me was not to turn this step into more stress. I wanted to get back into living my life after I rested of course, but I would take precautions. Early on, if I were traveling after a heavy adjustment morning, I'd sometimes take one Imodium and go on with my activities. This would decrease potential stress by putting my mind at ease and helping me not worry about the chance of recurrence. I generally did not like taking Imodium because it slowed down the important action of the probiotics, but in some rare circumstances during the healing process, it was necessary. Once I rested, it did my soul much good to get into some activity I enjoyed. It helped put the heavy adjustment behind me, and always made me look forward to a better tomorrow.

Before I hit my probiotic dosage goal, I learned to watch if the adjustment symptoms lasted for more than four days without some improvement. If so, this was most likely a sign that I could have gone up too fast in probiotics for the week. In either case, lowering my probiotic dosage for the week was the solution. I can't stress enough how important it is to listen to your own body.

Roadblock: Second-guessing Herxheimer reactions

Breakthrough: Once I understood that by sticking to my program I was not directly responsible for causing these Herxheimer reactions, I wasn't bothered by any brief uncomfortable moments if they did occur.

Early on in my program, when Herxheimer reactions were more common, I did have some challenging ones. Sometimes after the repeated bathroom trips, cramps and soreness. I felt totally exhausted. Then I started to think, "What did I eat? Was it too many nuts? Was it that wine I had on the weekend? Or did I get food poisoned?" Those are natural responses while being on my program, and a perfect example of what I call second-guessing a Herxheimer reaction. Unfortunately, it can make you frustrated if you let it, and that's why I call it a roadblock. It was a tough one too, until I found a better way to deal with it. Here's how I learned to lessen my second-guessing.

When I had a particularly heavy Herxheimer reaction, I tried not to get down on myself. I remembered that if I was following my diet correctly, I needed to stop thinking as if I cheated accidentally. That is just a recipe to become paranoid and add to stress levels. Ultimately, what helped me the most was reviewing the evidence from years of my daily journals. From the later successful trials, while formulating my program with the diet and probiotics, I concluded that occasional bad days are just the nature of the healing process and should not be misconstrued. These "bad days" are actually really good days – they are necessary adjustments (a.k.a. Herxheimer reactions) that my body needed to go through to bring my health to a higher level, so long as they didn't cause serious discomfort. (If so, it was wise to lessen the probiotic dose temporarily.)

My healing could not have occurred without building up the probiotic levels in my intestinal tract. An adjustment day occurs when an increase in the good bacteria from the probiotics pushes out the bad bacteria from the intestines; it's got to get out of the body to allow for healing. And this process often triggers symptoms that we may have had before like diarrhea, cramps, and occasionally for me, brief bleeding. So it's easy to think something is not working or to second-guess yourself and the diet. My journals showed that an adjustment to a probiotic increase could occur at any time during the week of the increase. Most often for me, it was within the first three days. The way I knew these adjustment days were not anything more serious was that even at their worst, they rarely lasted more than a couple of days.

One way I could tell that these adjustment days were helping me was that my overall concentration and energy would be increasing over time, most often every week or so. I did still experience them after I reached my probiotic dosage goal, but they lessened in their intensity and frequency as time went on. Once I understood that by sticking to my program I was not directly responsible for causing these adjustment episodes, I wasn't bothered by these occasionally uncomfortable moments when they did occur. I looked at them as my body doing what it had to do on the road to healing, and I was all for that.

Roadblock: Grumpy

Breakthrough: Go slow. Learn to be good to myself.

Journal entry from two months into Trial #8:

I've been having a rough time sleeping this week and it's tiring me out. Waking up in the middle of the night to go to the bathroom is so annoying! I'm cranky from not sleeping. I'm feeling impatient. And here I am again asking myself – is this illness ever going to go away? It's trying my patience today and I wish I could just wake up from this bad dream and go back to the way I used to be when I was well, when eating and bathroom trips weren't so all consuming.

Thoughts like these are completely normal even while being on the diet, especially in the beginning transition. Living with any illness, especially one that affects the gut, is extremely challenging. It would be a surprise if I didn't get moments of discouragement. But even though the temptation to be grumpy can be great, it won't do us any good to succumb to it; when we do, it can hurt our loved ones as well as ourselves. And you don't want to alienate the ones who love you, so here are some ideas for beating down grumpiness when it strikes.

I realize that losing sleep is a big factor in making me grumpier. And if I'm in a flare-up, a Herxheimer reaction, or battling a stomach bug - anything that makes my tough road more difficult - I'm even more susceptible to being grumpy. At times like these, I have to remember to give myself a break. I might ask for a little help from others, and I try to go easier on myself by not pushing to get too much accomplished. Most importantly, I recognize that I need more rest, preferably ASAP. This is the best thing I can do for myself when I'm grumpy. When my body tells me it's tired, I'll take a quick nap right away and get my strength back. It takes practice, but I find it almost impossible to be grumpy when I'm well rested.

Another trick of mine that also works here is to do exactly what I want at that moment. It works particularly well when I'm occasionally feeling worn down with the battle. Our lives are more challenging than most, so it's not hard to see that we should be a little more generous at being good to ourselves when we need it. I've seen it goes a long way. Other than healing, nothing keeps my positivity as high as enjoying a favorite pastime. Chances are I've been neglecting it, which could also be the reason why I'm feeling grumpy. Not denying myself this pleasure at these times makes me feel this illness can't stop me from living my life, and that makes the grumpiness subside. Thus, while healing it's critical not to lose sight of the fun I can have. If I've been waiting to go see a movie, then I go do it. Stop and read that book, go for a walk, play that video game, sit outside in the sun, draw a picture or whatever feels right, just not cheating on the diet. This really swings my spirit to the positive side, and my grumpiness disappears. It usually doesn't take long to feel great. Sometimes, I stop postponing playing the guitar, and just play it for fifteen minutes. Almost instantly, I forget what I was grumpy about, and I'm much happier to do whatever tasks I have left that day.

In the beginning of my program, a crucial part is one of transition. It's about modifying old behaviors that were not helping. I use these times when I'm grumpy as an excellent opportunity for growth, to teach myself to go slow and try not to fight the feelings of transition. In this way, I'm learning to help myself reach my goals, not keep myself from them.

PART 6: What I Gained

I made a choice to improve my health and was surprised by how much more I gained in doing so. Not only did my program help me recover, which alone is amazing, but I also reaped unexpected personal benefits that changed me more than just physically. Some of these came in the form of life lessons that many people never have the opportunity to learn. As you could imagine, I was surprised that my physical adversity became an opportunity for growth. Here are some of my favorite benefits that came to me while sticking with my program.

Control

Everyone wants it: to have control over their lives and the outcomes that affect them, but it's very hard for anyone to retain in this often-chaotic world. And we know all too well that it's even more difficult with an illness like IBD or IBS, which really becomes a daily reminder of our loss of control. Depression, sadness, anger and frustration usually result, and are all natural reactions to this loss. But *gaining control was not going to come by giving up.*

When I first started the diet, being restricted to only eating foods that would nourish me was something totally new. Unfortunately, I had many preconceived negative attitudes and I saw it as denying myself the snack food I loved. I could no longer seek the comfort of my favorite comfort foods. I was not allowed the "freedom" to eat whatever I wanted anymore. But in the hopes of helping myself, I chose to ignore those feelings of suffering and proceed. Surprisingly, after a short time, what I initially thought I was giving up, I was actually getting back! I was getting the control that had escaped me for so many years, the control I had always wanted over my body, and my life.

In a nutshell, this "restricted" diet was helping me get free again. Free from the toilet holding me prisoner, free from the endless worry about losing control, and free from having to plan my day around toilet locations. Believe me, when you start to get that freedom back, you realize that no food tastes as good as freedom feels. The diet was teaching me to make better food choices, as well as nourishing my body better than ever.

My program showed me that I was able to gain control in my life by controlling what I put in my mouth. It all starts there. Once I realized the benefit of gaining control this way, staying on the diet became easy. Early on after this epiphany I wrote, "I never want to get off the diet," and that was even before I really began healing!

My early trials showed that the right foods make me feel good and the wrong foods make me feel bad, it's just that simple. After realizing that, I didn't care how good bread or sugar tastes. I'd rather have my life back than an overrated, five-minute, taste-bud thrill ride. That is control. I proved to myself that the benefits of exerting control with my diet seep into all aspects of my life, making me a better, happier person. I became one who says, "I can" instead of "I can't," and witnessed dramatic improvement in my life.

Even people without IBD and IBS experience sadness when they feel out of control. Take a minute to reflect on what is making you sad now, and see if you can discover how it is rooted in control. You become free when you see that you always have a choice. It's as if you are riding a horse but you never look down. If you looked down, you'd see that you have the reigns in your hands; you are in control if you choose to be. Similarly, because you can choose, you really are in control of your life at all times. I like to remember that my life is an open road and I always have the reigns - always - I just need to notice that I do.

Freedom

Journal entry from two months into Trial #7:

My sister called to meet me for lunch today. I've already been to the bathroom and done my morning "business." My confidence is a little shaky because I haven't really tried going out much since I started the program, but I do feel good. Let's push it and see what happens today; I'm gonna go. It's at a place a half hour away. I think I can do it!

Afternoon journal entry from the same day:

Just got back from lunch, and would you believe, I feel great! No panic. No urgency. No cramps. No need for the bathroom. It feels like my life is being restored! This is awesome… can't believe I haven't had to go yet!

OH!! Forgot to mention that in the back of my mind, before I got to the restaurant, I was thinking that if I don't feel good, I could always come home right after lunch. But I brought my grocery list anyway, in the hope that I could go there after and save a trip. I felt so normal and strong after lunch that I decided to go to the grocery, then the pet store, and then finally home. For the first time since I almost can't remember, I did what I wanted when I wanted. Incredible! Bowel functions are going further back in my list of things to think about, that's the best! And this is only two months into my program. Freedom never tasted so good.

Positivity

Journal entry from four months into Trial #13:

Feels incredible to be getting well again. I just had to write today and try to describe it. I'm going through that new level of awakening again as I did in Trial #7; I can really see and feel improvements from days not so long ago. I had hoped I could repeat the success, but never thought that it would ever feel this good. What's really incredible is that while I'm slowly chipping away at becoming whole again, I'm treated with a new found sense of confidence and lust for life that has been absent in me for years. This life is loaded with so many fun things to do and think about, things I haven't been able to be part of for so long. It's hard to believe there was a time I felt I just couldn't go on. I feel just the opposite now.

I've gone from feeling like my life was a curse, and now it's a gift. The bad feelings and negative mindset that used to plague me are disappearing; I've never been so grateful. There's so much to see and do - even while I'm healing - and I can't wait to do more of it! It's overwhelming to think that I'd still be trapped where I used to be if I didn't try to find my program. Healing was so worth the effort.

Seeing the Big in the Small

I can't overemphasize how important celebrating each accomplishment was to me during my healing. It's a great practice I still use today to keep my spirit high. I like to say that *no success is too small to make a big deal out of*. It's like a snowball effect on your positivity, and naturally increases good times. On days when I realized I needed the bathroom less than the week before, I definitely shouted about it (to the laughs and delight of my family). When my guts started to feel strong and have that "normal" feeling like they used to, I went outside in the sun and just had a grateful moment to myself; my efforts had been validated! I sat in the sun and cultivated those good feelings in my body, letting it grow in my mind and heart, until I felt like my life was a celebration. Everybody's life can be, even while fighting an illness.

My eyes opened to the bigness in all the small moments and mundane tasks around me. In fact, most of our lives are full of these small moments. Many people don't see them because they've stopped noticing. I didn't want to do that anymore. When I was really sick I was also too busy to notice, but as I healed, these moments became obvious. I made it a point that I would no longer take them for granted, just as I did with my improvements in health. When you stop taking those moments for granted, you see how much potential joy you were missing out on daily. While I was healing it became clear: why waste time waiting for big moments to be joyful, when there are plenty of small moments to celebrate right now?

Nourishing My Body

Journal entry from three months into Trial #1:

I've naturally toned down my noshing habit (i.e., mindlessly munching on snacks) and have embraced eating a healthy balanced diet. Yes, I feel real good today. At first, I was still in my pretzel and chip noshing habit, and needed to replace them with something on the diet. It happened to be a nut mix I'd make. But I was eating too much, causing my gut to be sore. Now that I'm stopping this excessive nut binging, I'm reprogramming my mind's cravings, and it's working.

In fact, I needed this. My eating habits were bad: too many bad carbs and not enough good carbs, namely, fruits and veggies. I had no room for them, let alone respect. I couldn't nourish my body when my stomach was full of pretzels and chips. And it's not just me; it's an American epidemic. With record numbers of diabetes and obesity on the rise, it would seem that we just don't know how to eat right in this country. Bad habits get formed too easily. And they are only reinforced through the marketing efforts of food manufacturers to always tempt us.

If I didn't get colitis, I'm sure I would have eaten myself into some other life threatening illness. I'm happy today knowing that my program saved me from going down that road to ruin. I don't miss my old snack habits at all; if I still followed them, I couldn't feel this good now. That's why I always nourish my body when I eat.

Mind Over Sugar

Journal entry from six months into Trial #6:

I was in a drug store today waiting at the counter, and it dawned on me that I was surrounded by all my old favorite, quick-grab, sugary treats. Surprisingly, those treats weren't the first thing I noticed anymore. In fact, I really didn't "see" them at all. It was like they were invisible; they no longer had any power over me.

I was over the physical addiction of sugar and bread within sixty days. During which time I was forming a new mindset. It was as simple as recognizing that if I continued to be compelled by my cravings, I would never truly be free. At that point, I became turned-off whenever I saw those sweets and breads in any grocery store, gas station, or vending machine. Soon resisting them became a thrill instead of a challenge; it was easy! Every time I resisted, I received a greater sense of power. And it just snowballed. I was now in charge of my health, and that's when I just didn't feel those temptations anymore.

New Level of Cool

Journal entry from three months into Trial #7:

A quick note about how well I'm doing with all my personal challenges lately. It's a great example of how my program has helped my personal growth. I've gotten much better about staying cool, and going with the flow while enduring my worst personal times to date.

This week my brother and I have had to close our business because of the recession, and lack of work. Finding work elsewhere seems grim, as businesses everywhere are experiencing record layoffs. On top of that, I've been dealing with my divorce issues, like rushing to get this house on the market and all the work that it requires. I'm choosing and coordinating the contractors for necessary fix-ups. Dad and I have decided to do the landscaping. My wife and I are doing the interior painting and the demolition to a basement storage room because of a cracked main sink drain beneath the floor, perfect timing huh? Now I can't use the kitchen sink, so I've got to go to my sister's place in the next town to cook my food for the diet. And if that isn't bad enough, some days the plumbers shut off all the water, so I have to go to her house for the bathroom too. Best of all, I'm making it look easy, and I'm even in a flare-up now! That would have been impossible for me to handle, just three months ago.

I think back now about how I used to be and can't believe the changes I've made - and so quickly at that! I see that poor food choices would have been a false comfort to me at this time. It is my discipline that now provides the comfort for my body and spirit. My old eat-anything-I-please ways would have sabotaged me to a point of uselessness; I would've needed the toilet too much. That would just be unacceptable now. Too much has to be done. I have to be strong and make it through. My program showed me that when the going gets tough, don't succumb to comfort food, stay strong and persevere. It's so much better to feel useful instead of useless. To help myself instead of hurt myself. It is the act of staying focused and committed to my program that is granting me this freedom I enjoy now. I think the message here is loud and clear: even at the worst point in my life, I am not a loser, I am a winner.

All the Things You Can Do When You're Not on the Toilet

Journal entry from four months into Trial #7:

My brother's wedding in New York City this past weekend was fantastic. My new freedom made me love the city as never before – it was sheer joy! Got over the

Herxheimer reaction from the probiotic increase, and I was confident that I wouldn't have any emergencies. Using the pattern my body was showing from previous journal notes, I timed it so that I'd be strong for the trip, and I must say, I planned it perfectly. It was easy to stay on my diet too; I brought my baked cookies and ate lots of salmon and chicken with salad.

NYC is a much different place when you're not looking for the bathroom all the time. This trip had a message that was loud and clear to me: you don't have to be completely recovered to start enjoying more of what life has to offer. And to think, it's been just four months into this trial. So to prove that point, I set a personal record by seeing four rock shows over the weekend. I didn't force myself, I just had the opportunity. And for the first time, I felt well enough to do it. Who's got gut troubles? Doesn't feel like me!

Life tastes so good right now, even if I'm not completely healed yet. I can do things, such as take my time and just walk in the street and shoot photos in NYC - all the fun stuff I never had time to even consider before. I even started taking for granted that I was leaving the hotel room and not wondering if I was going to need a bathroom. A feeling I have sorely missed.

Noticed a new strength in my gut lately too, not so evident in the stools yet, but a new feeling of "solidness" from my body. I am really enjoying just eating a meal, and leaving the house. (Yes, one of the great underestimated joys of life!) And just like that, I'm off on another mission. I'm content because I went once in the AM, and (from reviewing journal notes) it's not likely I'll be going again. That's the big reason to remember why I don't cheat on the diet – so I can be reliable! That's where my confidence comes from.

So to celebrate my newfound freedom, I drove over to my guitar lesson, parked my car five blocks away, and walked to my teacher's house just to take in the sights. I could've parked closer, but now I didn't need to. After the lesson, I walked back to my car and then drove across town to see one of my favorite bands at a club. Finally, I was getting back to life instead of watching it from the sidelines; it felt incredible - just how I've wanted to live. It's what we all deserve. It didn't even matter much what I was doing, or where I was going, it was just the act of doing it that was the thrill. My mind was on my adventures again instead of always searching for a toilet.

To be around town and not have anxiety about my body for the first time since I got IBD was better than I ever dreamed!

It's a great reminder of how much I can do with my body when I'm well, and how much I was missing when I was really sick. Back then, I wasn't living a full life, but now I've got a second chance. I want to celebrate every new level of confidence and strength I get. This is why I worked so hard for years to find my program - now it feels like it was all worth it. It's what I always wanted: to be truly free and rid of that nasty second-guessing. Will I have to run to the bathroom again? Not anymore!

Lose the Comfort Foods, Find Yourself

Getting damaging comfort foods out of my life gave me the chance to finally focus on real self-improvement. It was the chance I needed for faster personal growth, free of distractions. Right away, my program showed me how much can be gained by denying myself these foods that used to make me feel so good. I have seen the benefits from re-thinking how I process bad feelings, bad luck, and bad days by not running to comfort food for a temporary "fix."

For me, comfort foods took away from my self-esteem, self-respect and kept me from my goals. "Oh, I'll figure that out tomorrow, but right now I'll have a pizza." It starts out harmless, then a habit is created, and it snowballs into a full-blown addiction that very few can resist. Food addiction is no different from any other addiction (alcohol, smoking, etc.). They're all the same. They feed on our weakness, they never say no, and ultimately, they keep us from reaching our true potential. How fast can you improve if you are always running for a fix?

I have gained so much time in my life by not being obsessed with getting comfort foods anymore, let alone the time spent eating them. I used to think about what crunchy, munchy, sugary thing I was going to eat next, even after I just finished one. Sometimes I'd go out of my way to go to a special store just for a favorite comfort food. It was easy to see how much time I was losing being obsessed with comfort food; it was hard to admit it.

My program changed all that. Suddenly, I didn't obsess about food anymore. I ate, nourished my body, and moved on. Best of all, I was on the toilet less! Suddenly, I had more time. I had more mental clarity, and ability to focus without distractions. My productivity increased. I had more time for "good" addictions, like physical exercise. And for this, I will always be grateful.

There are so many fantastic things to get into in life. I have learned that comfort food is not one of them. My program set me free to experience how great life can really taste, I would've never gotten here without it. It replaced the false confidence I got from comfort foods with a new sense of strength, and belief in myself. *It's amazing how much control I can have over my life when comfort food has no control over me.*

PART 7: What I Ate

Without even looking at my journal notes, I remember that my very first SCD™ meal in May '98 was breakfast. I had plain scrambled eggs. It was a bit of a departure from my usual bowl of sugary cereal, but it was also new, and really exciting to feel that I now had a hand in helping myself.

Since I went into the diet cold turkey, I didn't have any almond flour baked goods ready. Neither did I have many nutritious SCD™ choices available like fresh meat, fish, or fruits and vegetables. This was a house of bad carbs, sugar, and prepared food, but that was about to change. I was feeling a bit desperate, like clinging to a life preserver to the few diet safe items I had in my kitchen. I recognized that there were still many more that I couldn't have, like regular ketchup, which is loaded with sugar, for example. I was slowly making a transition in my head, and I liked having a plan, even though it felt a little strange to deny myself certain foods. On my second day of the diet, I remember cleaning out my cabinets of all remaining food products that were now off limits. It was time to start a new life, a new shopping list, and head to the grocery store with a new mindset. I didn't know what to expect, or how my body was going to react to the diet change.

What did happen was that I lost weight almost instantly. Even on the first day of the diet, I could feel my body being deprived of all the sugar and bread carbohydrates that I used to feed it, and it was not happy. I knew that the weakness and headaches I was experiencing on the second and third days were a withdrawal-type reaction from sugar and bread. By the fifth day I began to feel improvements in my guts, they felt so much less under siege; my whole body felt better. But I was still weak, and needed to start baking some almond flour bread and cookies right away to fill me up, and give me more energy. My sweet cravings were strong, so in the meantime I made sure to eat raisins, applesauce with cinnamon (no sugar added), and other gentle fresh fruits to satisfy.

122

Quickly, my body fell into a comfortable pattern of eating smaller meals more frequently. It felt natural. I had three main meals a day (breakfast, lunch and dinner), and a snack between each. I usually timed my last snack at night, around 8:30 PM, and that would most always carry me until morning.

Eating to Set the Stage for Healing

By keeping out the carbohydrates that my small intestine could not digest, I minimized the "food" source that the colon bacteria fed on. This allowed the probiotics to do their job of chasing out any pathogens and bad bacteria, as well as restoring the normal balance between intestinal bacteria. So, by following the diet, I set the stage for my healing. My trials were futile without it. It was also important to remember not to overdose on any particular food group. Eating balanced meals on the diet was critical to my nutrition, and my success.

My Typical Menus

Breakfast

Still the most important meal of the day! I was usually very hungry upon awakening since fasting from 9 PM the night before. All of my favorite menus are easy to prepare; here are some of my favorites that I rotate:

Option 1
Cheddar cheese pancakes (see Part 8, Favorite Recipes) with honey

Low sodium bacon or 100% natural breakfast sausage (neither with added sugar or starch)

Seasonal fresh fruit (My breakfast favorites are: grapefruit, melon, blueberries, raspberries, strawberries and very ripe bananas.)

100% natural OJ or Welch's 100% purple grape juice (I never drank my juices at full strength, I always diluted them (about 20% juice, 80% water) so they were easier on my stomach.)

Option 2

Egg sandwich (see Part 8, Favorite Recipes)

Fresh fruit

100% natural OJ or Welch's 100% purple grape juice

Option 3

(Almond flour) Congo Cookie Bar (see Part 8, Favorite Recipes)

One scrambled egg with cheddar cheese

Diet safe yogurt (see Part 8, Favorite Recipes) and fresh fruit

100% natural OJ or grape juice

Option 4

Two egg omelet (sometimes I made it from just egg whites) with peppers, onions, and Swiss cheese

Fresh fruit

Congo Cookie Bar

Lunch

Usually, lunch was a snap to prepare because I'd just reheat some tasty leftovers from dinner. That was one of the bonuses of making extra at dinner, and a good habit I got into quick. Most often I had what would be considered a small sized portion of salad, since a large portion was too hard on my gut. Also when I started the diet, I always favored cooked veggies to raw veggies. When I wasn't eating leftovers, these were some of my favorites:

Option 1

Salad with tuna from can (Packed in olive oil and salt only, like the Genova® Tonno brand. Absolutely no modified food starches.) I liked to include sliced cucumbers, carrots, tomatoes, cheddar, Swiss or havarti cheese, raisins and some of my nut mix (see Part 8, Favorite Recipes). I often used a commercial salad dressing, like Newman's Own® Olive Oil and Vinegar that I found with no added sugar or starch. If I were out, I'd just use my own olive oil with lemon, or red wine vinegar.

100% natural orange or grape "soda" (made from 20% natural juice and the rest club soda)

Option 2
Sandwich - on my focaccia bread (see Part 8, Favorite Recipes) with tuna salad (using homemade mayo made with no starch or sugar) or leftover chicken, pork, or lamb. I liked to include cheddar, Swiss or havarti cheese, lettuce, tomato, pickle and yellow mustard.

Squash chips (see Part 8, Favorite Recipes)

100% natural orange or grape "soda" (made from 20% natural juice and the rest club soda)

Option 3
Focaccia pizza - I'd split a slice of my focaccia bread in half, then top with homemade tomato sauce (no sugar or starch), peppers, onions, black olives, cheddar and jack cheeses, and a dash of Parmesan. If I had sausage that was sugar and starch free, I'd add that too!

Option 4
Cobb-style salad - I started with fresh tuna or chicken with cheddar cheese, bacon, olives, carrots, peppers, cucumbers, a handful of my nut mix, and olive oil and red wine vinegar. Umm! Umm!

Dinner

Dinner was always the main event. The more I experimented with TV cook show recipes and making the necessary diet substitutions, the more exciting dinner became. Every meal usually consisted of a protein (fish, chicken, pork or beef), a cooked vegetable, a small salad (if I wasn't experiencing a flare-up or a heavy Herxheimer reaction), some kind of almond flour bread or cookie, and/or fruit for dessert. Balanced meals like these always left me feeling satisfied.

I looked forward to summer because the outside grill seemed to make my entrées taste even better. I'd grill all sorts of fresh foods quickly like shrimp, sausages (containing no sugar or starch), chicken, pork, beef, fish etc.. Not only was there less to clean up, but when I'd call a bunch of friends over, there was nothing better. It was a favorite pastime, and one I could still do on my program, which did wonders for my spirit because I felt like one of the group - just hanging out and cooking on the grill!

In the beginning, I made simple entrées with only olive oil and a few herbs. This made things easy for me to know that everything was diet safe. From a cooking perspective, it also taught me how natural food really tastes. Very handy knowledge later on, when I wanted to choose the right herbs or spices for the seasoning of different meats, poultry and fish. Once I got comfortable with the diet, and I knew what I could and couldn't have, that's when the fun really started. There were many natural marinades, rubs, coatings and spice flavors I could devise to keep my taste buds happy, all while being diet safe. During the winter I didn't miss the barbeque too much with my George Foreman grill; it made my diet meals just as fast and delicious too. Another trick I learned was to make extra fresh cooked veggies and a salad at dinner, which would come in handy later in the week for fast leftovers.

I did my frying most often at dinner. I made a sensational fried haddock with just a simple egg and almond flour coating. On my frying nights, I would make an extra batch of squash chips to have for lunches and meals later in the week. Those were always great to have around - satisfying crunchy goodness!

At dinner, I almost always made a cooked vegetable. In the beginning, I used the frozen kind of approved veggies like peas, carrots and broccoli. But as my culinary skills improved, I much preferred the taste of fresh vegetables. My top picks are butternut squash, zucchini, broccoli, carrots, peppers, onions, celery and mushrooms. Often, I would finish each meal (if I was still hungry) with a small salad, and an almond flour cookie of some variety.

Marinated chicken, grilled or baked white fish, salmon, and pork tenderloin were among the entrées that I made frequently. I have too many favorites to list here, so I'll just mention a few: all types of fresh grilled fish with olive oil, fresh herbs, and sea salt, BBQ dry rub ribs (see Part 8, Favorite Recipes), almond flour pizza, parmesan encrusted chicken (see Part 8, Favorite Recipes), and of course, fried fish or shrimp with almond flour coating.

After I kicked my sugar addiction (about two months into the program), I found I craved fresh fruit following my dinner, and often preferred it to cookies. In my opinion, there's nothing like fresh cherries, raspberries or strawberries to cut the meal perfectly. Great for snacking during TV time too. (Go Sox!)

What I Ate During a Flare-up or Herxheimer Reaction

It was important for me to have a game plan when I went through early flare-ups, or heavy Herxheimer reactions. I knew that if I was experiencing soreness from these events, it was much better for me to lay off the nuts, raw vegetables, and raw fruits temporarily. Usually, if I cut them out for the rest of the day that I was sore, I could slowly resume them in small quantities the next day, only if feeling better. If that went well, I would return to my normal diet in another day or two.

Cooked vegetables and soft fruits became all the more important to eat when I cut out the raw ones. They would sustain me and provide necessary nutrients for my body to heal, and gently recover. So instead of having a salad with lunch or dinner, I'd have a small serving of cooked vegetables, or a desert of soft fruit. My favorites were very ripe bananas, and all-natural (no sugar added) applesauce. These always satisfied and sustained me well. When my stomach pain decreased, and my stools went back to the way they were before the upset or flare-up, I knew it was safe to start slowly adding my raw fruits and vegetables again.

What I Ate for Snacks

Early on, my almond flour Congo cookie bars (see Part 8, Favorite Recipes) were a perfect substitute for my comfort food snacks. But as I learned to enjoy the taste of fruits and yogurt, I soon realized that they too made an excellent snack, and provided more nutrients and variety as well. The more I mastered the diet, the more I used my snack time to include any food group, or vitamin rich foods, that I hadn't already with my meals. In this way, I was able to balance my daily nutrition nicely. Most often I enjoyed:

Option 1
Diet Safe Yogurt (see Part 8, Favorite Recipes) mixed with fresh fruit. Because of

my lactose intolerance, this was a critical source of my daily calcium, as well as providing the helpful probiotics. I made sure to get this everyday. To a half-cup of yogurt, I usually mixed in different combinations of fresh blueberries, strawberries, very ripe bananas, peaches, and a tablespoon and a half of honey. Yogurt was great anytime, but I most looked forward to it at night as my super satisfying last snack of the day.

Option 2
Homemade Nut mix and/or

Fresh quick-grab fruit (raisins, apple, very ripe banana, pear, peach or nectarine, etc.)

Option 3
Carrots and celery

Option 4
Cheese (cheddar, havarti, Swiss)

Olives

My focaccia bread with olive oil

Option 5
Congo Cookie Bar(s)

100% natural orange or grape juice (20% juice, 80% water or club soda)

Option 6
Fresh Fruit – applesauce (all natural, no sugar or starch added), raspberries, cantaloupe, and honeydew made an excellent dessert or snack. I also loved the quick-grab convenience of apples, very ripe bananas, and raisins.

The Joy of Variety

I'm always looking for new and exciting combinations of diet safe foods to satisfy. Creativity is key to the enjoyment of cooking and eating. Whether it's a snack, meal, or dessert, I understand that changing things up is essential to my happiness on any diet, and the SCD™ is no different. I knew that I was doing a good job about seeking out exciting recipes, and new twists on old stand-bys, because I never felt deprived on the diet.

It always amazes me when I stumble on a recipe, and it becomes my new favorite; I want to make it every week! That's why it's a good thing that these lists will never be "complete." I will always want to be adding and changing items to keep things interesting. You know how the saying goes, right? *Man cannot live on almond flour alone.*

PART 8: Favorite Recipes

Here are twelve great recipes that I still use all the time. Enjoy!

Focaccia bread

1½ cups Farmer's Cheese (a.k.a. Dry Curd cottage cheese)
5 eggs (three with yolks, and two just whites)
6 tablespoons melted butter
6 cups almond flour
1½ cups fine grated Parmesan cheese (no fillers or starch added)
1 teaspoon baking soda
1½ teaspoon salt
½ cup water

In a food processor, or a mixer (I think it comes out best in a food processor) add the eggs, butter, and Farmer's cheese. Start at low speed, and then blend just until you get a smooth, creamy texture. In a big mixing bowl, add the almond flour, Parmesan, baking soda, salt and mix briefly by hand. Add the creamy mixture from the food processor to the contents of the mixing bowl. Add the ½ cup water and fold with spatula or hands, just until it makes a consistent dough-like mass. Do not over handle!

Pre-heat oven to 325° F. Take an 11"x17"x1" rectangular baking pan, spray with canola spray, and add mixture. Spread to cover whole pan with hands (dip hands in water if needed), then use spatula dipped in a little water to make top smooth and even. Apply egg wash to top (beat one more egg, then brush on top) and sprinkle on oregano. Bake 15 minutes on bottom rack. Then switch to top rack for 15 more minutes. Use toothpick to test if done. Cook to golden brown (cooking time may vary depending on oven). Allow to cool. Cut square pieces evenly. Each piece can be cut in half to make sandwiches or toast.

Yield = 24 slices of focaccia bread

(Almond Flour) Congo Cookie Bars

½ cup canola oil
1 stick melted butter
1⅓ cups honey
1 teaspoon baking soda
1 teaspoon salt
2 cups raisins
1½ cups unsweetened coconut chips
8 cups almond flour
1½ tablespoons cinnamon (optional)
½ cup water

In a big mixing bowl, add all the ingredients except the almond flour and water. Mix well with spatula. Add 4 cups of almond flour and mix. Add the last four cups of almond flour and mix again. Add the water slowly while mixing in the last of the almond flour to make a smooth cookie dough-like texture, dough should feel thicker rather than thin. Pre-heat oven to 300° F.

Spray a 12"x18"x2" rectangular baking pan with canola spray. Spread in dough mixture and smooth with hands or spatula dipped in water. *Option 1:* with a plastic knife, gently score the dough surface, making small squares. Top each square with a half walnut, half pecan or almond if desired. *Option 2:* (carmel-like icing) in a mixer or foodprocessor, mix ½ cup butter, 1 cup honey and 3 teaspoons vanilla until smooth. Spread on top of dough in pan and sprinkle evenly with more unsweetened coconut chips.

Put in oven on bottom rack and bake for 15 minutes. Then switch to top rack and bake for another 15 minutes. Cookies are done when golden brown. (Oven temp and times may vary.) Test with toothpick for doneness. Let cool, cut into squares.

Yield = 60 cookies

Cheddar Cheese Pancakes

3 cups almond flour

3 eggs (I use jumbo eggs, one whole egg with it's yolk, and the whites of the two others)

3 tablespoons of honey (less if you don't like it sweet)

1 cup of yogurt (according to recipe later in this section)

½ teaspoon salt

½ teaspoon baking soda

2 dashes of canola oil

¼ cup water

1 cup fresh shredded real cheddar cheese (not from pre-shredded package, those contain starch)

In a medium/large mixing bowl, add all ingredients together except for cheddar cheese. Warm griddle between medium and medium low heat. (I like a big rectangular griddle, one that spans two heating elements.) Batter should be a smooth, flowing consistency, not thin like water, and not thick like cookie dough. (Add a touch more water and a dash more oil if needed.)

Spray griddle liberally with canola spray. Using a ¼ measure, pour ¼ cup of batter onto griddle and repeat, leaving room for each pancake to expand a little. Sprinkle a little cheddar cheese on top of each pancake. Let cook 4-5 minutes until underside of pancakes start to brown. Carefully flip and let cook another 2-3 minutes to a light golden brown. If batter thickens up between batches, just add a little water and whisk.

Variation: can also add bacon pieces (no sugar) with the cheddar cheese or blueberries. Serve with honey as "syrup."

Yield = approximately 20 small/medium size pancakes

Breakfast Egg Sandwich

1 egg
1 slice of focaccia

Optional:
sliced cheddar cheese
fresh salsa (no sugar or added starch)
fresh guacamole (no sugar or added starch)
bacon or sausage (no sugar or added starch)

Split a focaccia bread slice in two, and toast. Spray a medium/small microwave bowl with canola spray and crack a fresh egg into it. Cover with a paper towel and cook on high for about forty seconds. Coat the toast with fresh salsa, fresh guacamole, or a shot of your favorite hot sauce. Put the egg on one half of the toast, add cheddar cheese, some bacon or sausage, and top with the other half of toast.

Who's hungry?

Steve's Awesome Nut Mix

raw almonds
raw pecans halves
raw walnut halves
2 tablespoons canola oil
salt
honey

Pre-heat oven to 325° F. In a 11"x17"x1" rectangular baking pan, add even amounts of almonds, pecans and walnuts spread out evenly to form a relatively thin layer. Drizzle on the oil. Mix by hand to coat evenly, then spread them out to form a thin layer again. Salt lightly.

Bake on bottom rack for 12 minutes. Remove. Mix nuts with spatula. Lightly salt again. Bake on top rack for 10 minutes more or until the pecans are medium brown. Do not burn. Remove. Let cool for 5 minutes. Drizzle with honey and mix with spatula. (Salt again or drizzle with honey a second time if desired.)

Options: can add unsweetened coconut chips and raisins during honey process for a delicious trail mix. Also, can make a spicy version with diet-safe, all natural Cajun spice if you can find it. Experiment!

Armenian Style Burgers (a.k.a. "Losh" kebob)

1 pound lamb, beef, or turkey
1 medium chopped sweet onion
¼ cup chopped parsley
¼ cup chopped red pepper
¼ cup chopped green pepper
4 to 6 ounces tomato juice
1 teaspoon cumin
½ teaspoon cayenne pepper
salt and pepper

Mix all ingredients together, knead with hands. Moisten hands with water to help shaping. Form a patty shape with the meat mixture and grill on top of stove in non-stick pan sprayed with oil, or on barbeque grill.

Yield = 4 to 6 patties

Parmesan Encrusted Chicken

4 boneless skinless chicken breasts
¾ cup fresh coarse grated Parmesan cheese
black pepper
2 tablespoons olive oil

Rinse chicken breasts and dry on paper towels. Place grated Parmesan in a flat dish, sprinkle with fresh ground black pepper. Press the chicken into cheese mixture, on both sides.

In a large skillet over medium heat, add olive oil and the chicken breast and cook 5 to 8 minutes per side, depending on size of chicken breast. Remove to serving plate.

Big El's BBQ Ribs

1 tablespoon salt
1 tablespoon ground cumin
1 tablespoon black pepper
1 tablespoon chili powder
2 tablespoons paprika
2 to 4 pounds spareribs

Mix first five ingredients in a small bowl, blending together. Sprinkle the spices over the ribs and rub all over.

Place in roasting pan and roast at 300° F for an hour and half.
Check for doneness and continue baking if needed.

Taco-style Meat Filling

1 pound lean beef or turkey
1 teaspoon salt
1 teaspoon pepper
2 teaspoon chili powder
1 teaspoon cumin
1 teaspoon paprika

In a large skillet, sauté and mash meat to a fine size. Cook and stir until meat is done. Drain any excessfat and blot a little with paper towels. Now add spices and mix together under low heat until well blended. Serve as desired; try over vegetables or toasted focaccia. Great over salad, like tostada-style.

Ellie's Crab Cakes

1 pound lump crabmeat
½ small onion chopped fine
¼ cup chopped red pepper chopped fine
¼ teaspoon dried thyme
¼ teaspoon hot sauce (no added sugar or starch)
½ teaspoon salt
½ teaspoon pepper
5 to 6 tablespoons canola mayonnaise (no added sugar or starch)
3 tablespoons olive oil

Pull apart crabmeat and mash to a course consistency. Mix all ingredients, except olive oil, form and shape into whatever size patty desired.

Heat oil in a large skillet. When hot, add patties carefully and sauté over medium heat, 3 to 4 minutes on each side.

Steve's Chips (Fried Squash Chips)

2 medium to large butternut squash
canola oil
salt

Rinse and peel squash. Cut 2 inch sections. (For the bottom part with seeds, cut in half, scoop out seeds and then cut remaining squash in half.)

Heat up canola oil in home fryer. Use food processor with thin slicing blade (the thinner the blade, the crunchier the chips). Put squash sections into processor, and slice into thin slices. Load slices into fryer. Fry for 5 minutes, stir and turn chips with a grated metal frying spatula, and fry for another 5 minutes. Chips are done when golden brown. Remove and put chips in clean paper grocery bag, add a few dashes of salt, close and shake bag a few times to cover chips evenly. Allow chips to cool while you load next batch into fryer.

Yield = 20 – 30 oz. of chips

Diet Safe Yogurt (lactose, starch, and sugar free)

1 half-gallon 2% or whole milk (whole milk makes the yogurt more firm and tasty)
Natren® Yogurt Starter
home yogurt maker with liquid thermometer

In a medium sauce pan, heat milk *slowly* on medium low heat until temperature reaches 180° F. (Takes approximately 30-45 minutes.) Keep at that temperature for 5 minutes. Let cool to 115° F. (Takes approximately 40 minutes.)

Once the milk reaches 115° F, in the yogurt maker container add 1-2 teaspoons of the yogurt starter and about a ½ cup of the lukewarm milk. Stirring gently with whisk until starter is dissolved.

Add rest of milk slowly, stirring as you add. Cover and follow directions for your yogurt maker, *but then allow it to stay undisturbed for 24 hours.* (This is how the yogurt becomes lactose and sugar free.) Remove after 24 hours and refrigerate immediately.

PART 9: Good Problems to Have

In my tenth month of both successful Trials #7 and #13, I became acutely aware of my improved health. So much so, that I forgot I was ever really sick. One night, while at dinner out, the bread was being passed and I almost reached out to try it. I had never done that before - I was shocked - mostly because it felt so natural. It's not like I was tempted, I was well accustomed to the diet, but maybe subconsciously my body felt so healthy that it didn't recognize I had any special diet needs. Of course, I caught myself before I made a mistake and cheated, and I just chalked it up to the fact that my program was indeed working. It was a natural reaction that I never anticipated, but it was time to face it. The moment had come. I now had to deal with feeling good.

Was temptation now going to strike in a new way? I felt so good, could I handle a taste of this, or a snitch of that? I wondered. I referred back to *Breaking the Vicious Cycle* where Elaine recommended to follow the diet for at least one more year after all symptoms have gone. That sounded like a good plan and one I knew I could handle. After all, I know what got me here.

By remembering to focus on the time I'm having and not forbidden food, I kept myself from falling back into my old habits. This was my highest point of health yet; one I couldn't even dream of less than a year ago. It was time to celebrate the fact of this new milestone, just not with forbidden food. I've worked too hard to forge new eating routines that nourish my body, and have given me all the freedom that I now enjoy. It would be foolish to throw all that progress away.

That's when I realized that *my program isn't about going back to what I was used to, it's about being better than I ever used to be.* And I'll continue doing it by keeping up with what got me here, and finding comfort in knowing that it's proven. They'll be plenty of time for snitching a sample of some forbidden food when the time comes, but I wouldn't trade feeling this good for anything. All I have to do is remember how sick I was before my program, and I have my proof: these really are good problems to have.

GLOSSARY

Antibiotic
A substance that kills or inhibits the growth of living microorganisms, like bacteria.

Bacteria
Microorganisms - either friendly or disease causing. Friendly bacteria normally present in the body protect against harmful invading organisms.

Bifidobacterium
Friendly bacteria that is present in the large intestine.

Carbohydrates
Food made up of sugars, starches, or fibers.

Complex carbohydrates
Food made up of fibers and/or starches.

Disaccharides
Sugars made up of two molecules chemically combined and require digestion before they can be absorbed into the blood stream. An example is table sugar, which is separated into glucose and fructose for digestion.

Enzymes
Proteins that act as a catalyst to speed up chemical reactions aiding digestion. Example: the enzyme sucrase catalyzes the reaction to split sucrose (digestion) into two single molecules, which are then absorbed into the blood stream.

Fibers
An indigestible carbohydrate found in some foods. Many molecules chemically combined.

Herxheimer reaction
Referring to a short-term immunological reaction to treatment in which the body experiences an increase in previous symptoms. Thought to be a result of harmful bacteria dying off.

IBD (Inflammatory Bowel Disease)
The name given to a group of disorders that cause the intestines to become inflamed. Examples are: Crohn's disease, and ulcerative colitis.

IBS (Irritable Bowel Syndrome)
An intestinal problem where food moves too quickly, or too slowly through the digestive tract.

Junk Food
Food that has low nutritional value, typically needing little or no preparation. Examples of which are processed snack foods and fast foods like burgers, fries, and sodas, which have been linked to obesity. Also see Pathogens.

Lactase
An enzyme that digests lactose.

Lactose

A disaccharide sugar present in milk. Digestion products are glucose and galactose.

Lactobacillus acidophilus

Friendly bacteria naturally present in the small intestine that protect it from invading harmful bacteria.

Lactobacillus bulgaricus

Friendly bacteria found in yogurt. As it passes through the body, it aids the activity of Lactobacillus acidophilus, and Bifidobacterium bifidum.

Mindfulness

Being aware of your present moment.

Monosaccharides

Simple sugars; single molecules that are immediately absorbed into the blood stream. There are three: glucose, fructose and galactose.

Pathogens

Disease carrying organisms. An example would be E.coli 0157:H7. In his bestseller, *Fast Food Nation*, Eric Schlosser points out that, "…Recent studies have found that many food borne pathogens can precipitate long-term ailments including IBD."

Polysaccharide

Many molecules chemically combined. Example foods are: rice, corn, potato, banana, and wheat.

Probiotics

Refers to friendly bacteria that live in the gastrointestinal tract.

Resistant starch

Polysaccharides that are resistant to enzyme action therefore undergo limited digestion. Example: unripe banana. These foods are partially digested in the colon and contribute to bacterial overgrowth. Conversely, a ripe banana is digestible.

Starch

A polysaccharide that is made up of lots of glucose molecules. Some are easily digested to glucose and some are not, such as an unripe banana.

ORDER FORM

GUT HELP:
GUIDE TO BREAKING FREE OF IBD AND IBS

(can also be ordered online at: **www.guthelp.com**)

USA (Continental)

	Total to Enclose
Price per book	$19.95
Florida residents add 6.5% sales tax.	$ 1.30
Add $4.50 for postage and handling for 1 book	$ 4.50 plus 50¢ for each additional book
(Add $.50 for postage and handling for each additional book.)	

Please complete the following and mail to: MAHAMA PUBLISHING, 14545 J Military Tr. #130, Delray Beach, FL 33484-3781

QUANTITY	PRICE	AMOUNT (quantity x price)
	$19.95	
	Subtotal	
	Florida Residents Add 6.5% Sales Tax	
	Postage and Handling	
	Total Enclosed *(Make checks payable to Mahama Publishing)*	

Name: _____

Address: _____

City/Town: _____ State: _____ Zip Code: _____

Thank You for your order!

Questions? Please email: info@mahamapub.com